Intermittent Fasting for Women Over 70

A Comprehensive Guide For Women To Learn Why Starting Fasting Is Never Too Late | Includes Simple and Tasty Recipes, a Meal Plan, an Exercise Plan & a Journal Diary

By

Melinda Francis

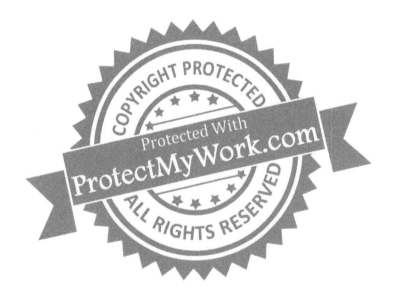

Table of Contents

Introduction

The golden years have arrived, and as women cross the threshold into their seventh decade, they bring with them a lifetime of experiences, wisdom, and a profound understanding of self. This stage of life is marked by the pursuit of happiness, contentment, and a sense of peace. Yet, like every chapter in life, it comes with its own set of challenges and changes that can impact the well-being and vitality of women over 70.

As we age, our bodies undergo natural transformations. It's no secret that, on average, women tend to gain weight after reaching the age of 60. Weight management becomes a prevailing concern, partly attributed to the replacement of lean muscle tissue with fat. The power to shape these transitions lies, to a significant extent, in the choices we make regarding our diet and lifestyle.

Weight loss, for many women over 60, can be an uphill battle, primarily due to the gradual slowdown of metabolism. The rate at which we burn calories decreases with age, but there's hope. By maintaining and even increasing lean muscle mass, we can influence the pace of the aging process. Intermittent Fasting (IF), a lifestyle choice rather than a restrictive diet, emerges as a powerful tool in this journey of self-care.

Intermittent fasting has garnered growing attention in recent years, not only for its potential to facilitate weight management but also for its array of health benefits that extend beyond the scale. It offers a flexible approach to eating, emphasizing when to eat rather than what to eat. It can enhance metabolism, promote mental well-being, and, intriguingly, may contribute to the prevention of certain age-related conditions, including specific nerve, muscle, and joint disorders.

IF's benefits are manifold, especially for women in their 70s. It has been linked to improved insulin sensitivity, resulting in reduced blood sugar and fasting insulin levels—critical factors in the battle against type 2 diabetes, a concern that often looms larger as we age. Studies suggest that IF can also mitigate inflammation, a driver of chronic diseases, and reduce cholesterol levels, a significant contributor to heart disease.

Beyond the physical advantages, intermittent fasting has a profound impact on mental health. It stimulates brain chemicals that promote cognitive clarity and may even aid in the preservation of brain function, an essential consideration in this phase of life.

In this book, we will delve into the principles, methods, and practicalities of intermittent fasting, tailored specifically to the needs and aspirations of women over 70. Together, we will explore how this approach can be your trusted companion in embracing your 70s with confidence, health, and a renewed sense of vitality.

Welcome to a journey of self-discovery and well-being. Your golden years are yours to embrace, and intermittent fasting is here to help you do just that.

Chapter 1: Unlocking the Power of Intermittent Fasting

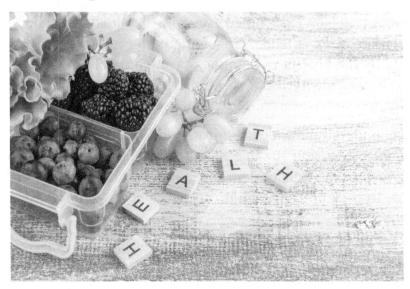

1.1 Fundamentals Of Intermittent Fasting And Its Potential To Transform Health

Intermittent Fasting is a lifestyle choice that has the potential to redefine your approach to health and well-being, especially as a woman in your 70s. At its essence, intermittent fasting is not just another diet trend; it's a deliberate way of structuring your eating habits. Unlike traditional diets that often impose strict food restrictions, IF focuses on when you eat rather than what you eat. It's about aligning your meals with specific time intervals, creating cycles of eating and fasting. Understanding the fundamentals of intermittent fasting is the first step toward unlocking its potential benefits.

The Timing of Meals. Intermittent fasting is centered around the principle of meal timing, a departure from the conventional focus on what you eat. It emphasizes not only the nutritional quality of your food but also when you consume it. This fundamental shift in perspective is what makes intermittent fasting a unique approach to nutrition and health for women over 70.

Metabolic Benefits. One of the most compelling advantages of intermittent fasting is its remarkable influence on metabolism. While intermittent fasting is often associated with weight loss, its benefits extend far beyond shedding a few pounds. As women progress into their seventies, the importance of metabolic health becomes increasingly evident. Thankfully, intermittent fasting has the potential to bring about profound metabolic changes that can significantly enhance overall well-being, potentially improving blood sugar control and insulin sensitivity. These metabolic benefits are of particular significance as we age and seek to maintain our health.

Weight Management. While weight loss is a common goal, intermittent fasting focuses on optimizing fat metabolism rather than just reducing body weight.

This approach can help women maintain a healthy body composition, preserving essential muscle mass and supporting a robust metabolism.

Mental Clarity and Focus. Intermittent fasting offers benefits that extend beyond the physical realm; it can have a remarkable impact on your mental clarity and cognitive function. Research suggests that intermittent fasting may stimulate the production of brain-derived neurotrophic factor (BDNF), a protein that supports the growth and maintenance of nerve cells. This can potentially lead to improved cognitive function, including enhanced memory, concentration, and mental clarity. Moreover, some individuals report improved mood and emotional stability while practicing intermittent fasting. This can be attributed to various factors, including the regulation of blood sugar levels and the release of feel-good neurotransmitters like serotonin. Intermittent fasting can also play a role in slowing down the aging process of the brain and providing neuroprotection.

Customizing Intermittent Fasting. Within the realm of intermittent fasting, there is a spectrum of approaches, each with its own nuances. The key is to discover the tailored approach that harmonizes seamlessly with your lifestyle and aligns with your personal health and wellness objectives. It's about finding the perfect equilibrium that complements your individuality.

1.2 The Science Behind Fasting

As we have already said, Intermittent fasting is not a trend; it's a scientifically grounded approach to optimizing your health, particularly as a woman over 70. To truly understand its potential, we need to venture into the world of scientific exploration, where the remarkable effects of fasting on aging and longevity are unveiled.

The Cellular Reset: Autophagy. At the core of intermittent fasting lies a fascinating process called autophagy. This term might sound complex, but its implications are profound, especially for women in their golden years. Autophagy is the body's natural mechanism for cellular renewal and repair. Imagine your body as a finely tuned machine. Over time, like any machine, it accumulates wear and tear. Cells become damaged, and waste materials accumulate. Autophagy is your body's way of performing maintenance, like a diligent mechanic. It clears out the damaged components, recycles them, and paves the way for the creation of new, healthy cells. What does this mean for you, the woman over 70? It signifies a potential reversal of the aging process at the cellular level. Intermittent fasting is like a trigger that activates autophagy, allowing your body to shed its old, worn-out cells and replace them with fresh, rejuvenated ones. This process can contribute significantly to your vitality and overall well-being.

Metabolism, Hormones, and Lean Muscle: The Key Players. Beyond autophagy, intermittent fasting influences fundamental aspects of your biology, including metabolism and hormone regulation. As we age, our metabolism tends to slow down, making it more challenging to maintain a healthy weight and energy levels. IF can help address this concern. Moreover, intermittent fasting affects hormones such as insulin and growth hormone. Insulin sensitivity, a crucial factor in blood sugar control, can improve through IF. This is particularly beneficial for women over 70, as it can help mitigate the risk of type 2 diabetes, a condition that becomes more prevalent with age.

Additionally, IF can play a role in preserving lean muscle mass, which is essential for strength and mobility as you age. By enhancing muscle retention, you can maintain your independence and overall quality of life.

A Closer Look at the Science. The science behind fasting is continually evolving, and researchers are uncovering new insights into its multifaceted benefits. We'll delve deeper into these aspects in the chapters ahead, providing you with a comprehensive understanding of how intermittent fasting can serve as a powerful ally in your journey toward improved health, longevity, and vitality.

Note: The long-term effects of intermittent fasting on weight loss for women are yet to be fully explored. While intermittent fasting is likely to aid in weight loss, individual results may vary depending on calorie consumption during non-fasting periods and adherence to the lifestyle.

1.3 Intermittent Fasting Methods Tailored To The Needs Of Women Over 70

Understanding the various intermittent fasting methods is key to finding the approach that aligns best with your lifestyle and health objectives.

1. The 16/8 Method

For many women over 70, simplicity is key. The 16/8 method is a popular starting point. It involves fasting for 16 hours and restricting your eating to an 8-hour window. For example, you might fast from 8:00 PM to 12:00 PM the next day, essentially skipping breakfast. For many women over 70, this approach can be particularly appealing because it allows you to align your fasting window with your natural circadian rhythms. This method may help regulate blood sugar levels, improve insulin sensitivity, and promote fat loss.

Advantages of the 16/8 Method

- ✓ **Simplicity:** The 16/8 method is easy to understand and follow, making it an excellent choice for beginners and individuals seeking a straightforward approach to intermittent fasting.

- ✓ **Alignment with Circadian Rhythms:** This method allows you to synchronize your fasting period with your body's natural circadian rhythms, potentially enhancing its effectiveness.

- ✓ **Blood Sugar Regulation:** Some research suggests that the 16/8 method may help regulate blood sugar levels and improve insulin sensitivity, which can be especially beneficial for those concerned about metabolic health.

- ✓ **Potential Fat Loss:** By restricting your eating to an 8-hour window, you create a calorie deficit that can contribute to fat loss over time, provided you make healthy food choices during the eating window.

Disadvantages of the 16/8 Method

- ✗ **Long Fasting Period:** A 16-hour fasting window may feel challenging for some individuals, especially if they are not accustomed to extended periods without food. It may require an adjustment period.

- ✗ **Skipping Breakfast:** The 16/8 method typically involves skipping breakfast, which might not be suitable for those who enjoy morning meals or have specific dietary preferences.

- ✗ **Individual Variability:** Intermittent fasting approaches can affect individuals differently, and what works for one person may not work as effectively for another. It's essential to monitor your body's response and make adjustments accordingly.

- ✗ **Potential Overeating:** During the 8-hour eating window, there's a risk of overeating or making less healthy food choices, which could negate the benefits of fasting. It's crucial to maintain balanced and nutritious meals.

2. The 5:2 Approach

Another approach that resonates with some is the 5:2 method. Here, you eat your regular diet for five days a week and restrict calorie intake to around 500-600 calories on the remaining two non-consecutive days. This method offers flexibility and can be adapted to your schedule. It can be an excellent choice for those looking to achieve health benefits without the commitment of daily fasting.

Advantages of the 5:2 Approach

- ✓ **Flexibility:** The 5:2 method provides flexibility, as it allows you to eat your regular diet for five days a week. This can be appealing to individuals who want to integrate intermittent fasting into their lives without the need for daily fasting.

- ✓ **Potential Health Benefits:** Research suggests that the 5:2 approach can offer various health benefits, including weight loss, improved insulin sensitivity, and reduced risk factors for chronic diseases.

- ✓ **Simplicity:** The concept of eating regularly for five days and restricting calories for two non-consecutive days is relatively straightforward and easy to follow.

- ✓ **Adaptability:** You can choose which days to designate as your low-calorie days, making it adaptable to your schedule and personal preferences.

Disadvantages of the 5:2 Approach

- ✗ **Hunger on Fasting Days:** On fasting days, calorie intake is significantly reduced (around 500-600 calories), which may lead to increased hunger and discomfort for some individuals.

- ✗ **Compliance Challenges:** Sticking to the restricted calorie intake on fasting days can be challenging, and some people may find it difficult to maintain.

- × **Potential Nutrient Gaps:** With reduced calorie intake on fasting days, there's a risk of not getting essential nutrients. It's crucial to ensure that the meals consumed on these days are nutrient-dense.

- × **Individual Variability:** As with any fasting approach, individual responses can vary. While some find success with the 5:2 method, others may not achieve the desired results.

3. The Eat-Stop-Eat Method

This method involves occasional 24-hour fasting periods, typically once or twice a week. It can be particularly effective for those who prefer fewer fasting days but with more extended fasting durations. It's essential to stay well-hydrated during these fasting periods.

Advantages of the Eat-Stop-Eat Method

- ✓ **Infrequent Fasting:** With the Eat-Stop-Eat method, you have occasional 24-hour fasting periods, typically once or twice a week. This means fewer fasting days compared to daily fasting approaches.

- ✓ **Extended Fasting Periods:** This method allows for longer fasting durations, which may provide additional benefits like enhanced fat burning and cellular repair.

- ✓ **Simplicity:** The concept of fasting for 24 hours once or twice a week is straightforward and easy to understand.

- ✓ **Autophagy and Cellular Repair:** Longer fasting periods can potentially stimulate autophagy, a cellular cleanup process that removes damaged components, contributing to overall cellular health.

Disadvantages of the Eat-Stop-Eat Method

- × **Hunger and Discomfort:** Fasting for a full 24 hours can lead to increased hunger and discomfort, especially on fasting days.

- × **Adherence Challenges:** Some individuals may find it difficult to adhere to the 24-hour fasting periods, and compliance can be a challenge.

- × **Nutrient Intake:** Extended fasting periods can increase the risk of nutrient deficiencies if meals are not properly balanced and nutrient-dense.

- × **Individual Variability:** As with any fasting approach, individual responses can vary, and what works well for some may not be suitable for others.

4. Alternate-Day Fasting

Alternate-day fasting, as its name implies, operates on a pattern of alternation between fasting days and regular eating days. During fasting days, calorie intake is notably reduced, creating a significant calorie deficit. On the flip side, regular eating days provide you with the freedom to consume your typical meals without restriction. This approach to intermittent fasting introduces a structured rhythm to your dietary routine. On fasting days, the reduced calorie intake prompts your body to tap into its energy reserves, ultimately contributing to weight management. It's essential to note that alternate-day fasting can vary in intensity, with some individuals opting for a complete fast on fasting days, while others allow for a limited caloric intake.

Advantages of Alternate-Day Fasting

✓ **Structured Rhythm:** Alternate-Day Fasting introduces a structured rhythm to your dietary routine, making it easier to adhere to a fasting schedule.

✓ **Calorie Deficit:** On fasting days, the reduced calorie intake creates a significant calorie deficit, which can contribute to weight management and fat loss.

✓ **Flexibility:** Alternate-Day Fasting can vary in intensity, allowing individuals to choose between a complete fast on fasting days or a limited caloric intake. This flexibility can suit different preferences.

✓ **Metabolic Benefits:** Some research suggests that alternate-day fasting may lead to metabolic improvements, including better insulin sensitivity and blood sugar control.

Disadvantages of Alternate-Day Fasting

✗ **Hunger and Discomfort:** Fasting days can be challenging due to increased hunger and potential discomfort from calorie restriction.

✗ **Compliance:** Strict adherence to alternate-day fasting may be difficult for some individuals, and it may not fit well with social or lifestyle commitments.

✗ **Nutrient Intake:** On fasting days, there's a risk of not meeting nutrient requirements, so it's crucial to plan balanced meals on regular eating days.

✗ **Individual Variability:** As with any fasting method, individual responses vary, and what works for one person may not be suitable for another.

5. The Warrior Diet

The Warrior Diet is a fasting method that stretches your fasting period to a remarkable 20 hours, leaving you with a concise 4-hour eating window typically in the evening. This approach often resonates with individuals who relish hearty evening meals and find comfort in the idea of fasting during the day. During the extended fasting period, your body has an opportunity to access stored energy reserves, promoting fat utilization and potential weight management. This method's distinct feature is the focus on consuming a substantial meal during the evening hours, which can offer a sense of satisfaction and fulfillment. What's crucial to understand is that there's no one-size-fits-all approach to intermittent fasting. Your lifestyle, preferences, and health considerations play a significant role in choosing the right method. Some may find daily fasting windows more manageable, while others may prefer occasional longer fasts.

Advantages of The Warrior Diet

✓ **Extended Fasting Period:** The Warrior Diet extends the fasting period to 20 hours, which allows your body to access stored energy reserves, potentially promoting fat utilization and weight management.

✓ **Satisfaction:** Consuming a substantial meal during the evening hours can offer a sense of satisfaction and fulfillment, especially for those who enjoy hearty evening meals.

✓ **Flexible Eating Window:** The 4-hour eating window in the evening provides flexibility for meal planning and social activities during the day.

Disadvantages of The Warrior Diet

- ✗ **Extended Fasting:** The 20-hour fasting period may be challenging for some individuals, leading to increased hunger and discomfort during the day.

- ✗ **Social Implications:** The Warrior Diet may not align well with social eating patterns, as the main meal is typically consumed in the evening.

- ✗ **Nutrient Timing:** Ensuring balanced nutrition within the 4-hour eating window is crucial, and some may find it difficult to meet their nutritional needs during this limited timeframe.

- ✗ **Individual Variability:** The Warrior Diet, like other fasting methods, may not be suitable for everyone. Individual preferences and lifestyle considerations should guide your choice.

1.4 Expert Guidance On Safely Initiating And Sustaining Intermittent Fasting

Embarking on your intermittent fasting journey is an exciting and empowering step towards better health. However, it's essential to approach it with caution, especially as a woman over 70. Here, we provide expert guidance to help you initiate and sustain intermittent fasting safely.

1. Consultation with a Healthcare Professional. Before beginning any fasting regimen, it's advisable to consult with your healthcare provider. They can assess your overall health, address any specific medical concerns, and offer personalized recommendations tailored to your needs.

2. Start Gradually. For those new to intermittent fasting, it's essential to ease into the practice. Begin with a less restrictive fasting schedule and gradually extend fasting periods as your body adapts. This approach minimizes the risk of discomfort or adverse effects.

3. Stay Hydrated. Proper hydration is crucial throughout your fasting periods. Water, herbal teas, and infusions can help maintain adequate hydration levels. Ensure you consume sufficient fluids to prevent dehydration.

4. Monitor Your Body. Listen to your body's signals. If you experience extreme hunger, dizziness, or other discomforts, it may be a sign to adjust your fasting schedule or consult with a healthcare professional.

5. Balanced Nutrition on Eating Days. On non-fasting days, prioritize a balanced diet that provides essential nutrients. Lean protein, whole grains, fruits, vegetables, and healthy fats are vital components of your meals. Consult with a nutritionist for guidance on a nutritionally sound eating plan.

6. Consider Supplements. As we age, our bodies may have different nutritional requirements. It's worth discussing with your healthcare provider whether you need any supplements to ensure you meet your nutritional needs during intermittent fasting.

7. Mindful Eating. Integrate mindful eating practices into your routine. Pay attention to hunger and fullness cues, savor each bite, and create a positive and intentional relationship with food.

8. Emotional Support. Fasting can sometimes trigger emotional responses. Seek emotional support from friends, family, or support groups if needed. Addressing the emotional aspect is essential for a holistic well-being journey.

9. Medication and Medical Conditions. For women over 70 who have medical conditions or are taking medications, it's essential to discuss intermittent fasting with their healthcare provider. Some medications may require adjustments to fasting schedules, and healthcare providers can provide guidance on managing health conditions while fasting safely.

10. Bone Health. Adequate calcium and vitamin D intake are crucial for maintaining bone health, especially for older women. Ensure your eating days include dairy products, leafy greens, and fortified foods.

11. Digestive Health. Digestive issues can become more common with age. Pay attention to how your body responds to fasting, and if you experience discomfort, consider adjusting your fasting duration or speaking with a healthcare provider.

12. Gentle Exercise. Incorporate gentle exercises like walking, yoga, or tai chi into your routine. These activities can complement intermittent fasting and promote overall well-being.

13. Sleep Hygiene. Quality sleep is crucial for overall health. Ensure you maintain a consistent sleep schedule and create a restful sleeping environment.

14. Stress Management. Managing stress is vital for health. Engage in stress-relief practices like meditation, deep breathing, or hobbies you enjoy to support your overall well-being. Remember that intermittent fasting should enhance your health and not cause undue stress. It's a flexible and adaptable approach, and it's okay to modify it to suit your comfort and needs.

1.5 Expert Advice on Maintaining Safety and Well-being Throughout the Process

As you continue your journey with intermittent fasting, it's essential to prioritize safety and well-being, especially as a woman over 70. Expert advice can guide you in this aspect.

1. Hydration Continues to Be Key. Maintaining proper hydration remains crucial throughout your intermittent fasting journey. Ensure you drink an adequate amount of water, herbal teas, and hydrating liquids to support overall health.

2. Regular Monitoring. Continue monitoring your body's response to intermittent fasting. Pay attention to any discomfort or unusual symptoms and adjust your fasting schedule accordingly.

3. Consistency Matters. Consistency is key to success in intermittent fasting. Stick to your chosen fasting schedule as closely as possible to help your body adapt and optimize the benefits.

4. **Mindful Eating Remains Important.** Mindful eating practices, which we discussed earlier, continue to be relevant. Pay attention to portion sizes and the quality of your food on non-fasting days to maintain balanced nutrition.

5. **Support Network.** Lean on your support network, whether it's friends, family, or support groups. Sharing your intermittent fasting journey can provide encouragement and motivation.

6. **Stay Informed.** Keep yourself informed about the latest research and information regarding intermittent fasting for women over 70. Staying up-to-date allows you to make informed decisions.

7. **Periodic Health Check-ins.** Schedule regular health check-ups with your healthcare provider. These check-ins can help you track your progress and ensure that intermittent fasting aligns with your overall health goals.

8. **Holistic Well-being.** Remember that well-being encompasses physical, mental, and emotional health. Prioritize self-care, stress management, and maintaining a positive outlook as part of your holistic approach to well-being.

1.6 Inspiring Success Stories of Women Who Have Embraced This Approach

Within the pages of this book, we have the privilege of sharing with you a collection of remarkable success stories. These stories are a testament to the transformative potential of intermittent fasting for women over 70. While the stories featured here are just a glimpse into the thousands of success stories that exist, they hold the power to inspire and illuminate the possibilities that lie ahead. You probably know that I am Melinda Francis, a nutritionist, and the women whose journeys you will read about are not only my patients, but they are also individuals who have generously chosen to share their personal experiences. These stories offer a glimpse into the real-life impact of intermittent fasting on the lives of women over 70, showcasing the resilience, determination, and vitality that can be achieved through this approach. As you read through these narratives, I hope you find inspiration and insights that resonate with your own journey toward improved health and well-being. Each story is a testament to the potential for positive change, and it is our sincere hope that they empower you to embrace the possibilities that intermittent fasting can bring to your life.

Ellen's Story: Rediscovering Vitality at 72. Ellen, a vibrant 72-year-old, struggled with weight gain and fatigue in her later years. After learning about intermittent fasting, she decided to give it a try. With guidance from her healthcare provider, Ellen embarked on a 16/8 fasting schedule. Over time, she noticed increased energy levels, improved mental clarity, and steady weight loss. Ellen's success story is a testament to how intermittent fasting can help older women regain vitality.

Grace's Journey: Managing Diabetes and Thriving at 68. Grace, at the age of 68, was living with type 2 diabetes. Her journey with intermittent fasting began after consulting her healthcare team. By incorporating a tailored fasting plan, she achieved remarkable improvements in her blood sugar control.

Grace's success demonstrates the potential of intermittent fasting to manage age-related health conditions.

Margaret's Transformation: Embracing a Healthier Lifestyle at 75. Margaret, at 75, was determined to age gracefully. She adopted intermittent fasting as part of her holistic approach to well-being. Alongside her healthcare provider's advice, she followed a 5:2 fasting regimen. Margaret's journey led to not only weight loss but also enhanced mental focus, reduced inflammation, and a newfound sense of well-being. Her story illustrates the power of intermittent fasting for overall health.

Jane's Resilience: Thriving at 71 Through Fasting. At 71, Jane faced age-related challenges, including muscle loss and reduced metabolism. She incorporated intermittent fasting into her life with the guidance of a registered dietitian. Jane's commitment to the 5:2 fasting method resulted in improved muscle mass maintenance and metabolic function. Her story is a testament to the resilience that intermittent fasting can instill in older women.

Evelyn's Wellness Transformation at 74. Evelyn, a vibrant 74-year-old, had been struggling with arthritis and joint pain. She decided to explore intermittent fasting to see if it could help. With guidance from her healthcare provider, Evelyn adopted a 12-hour time-restricted eating window. Over time, she noticed reduced inflammation, improved joint mobility, and an overall boost in her well-being. Evelyn's story highlights how intermittent fasting can support joint health in older women.

Linda's Journey to Heart Health at 69. Linda, at the age of 69, had concerns about her heart health due to a family history of heart disease. She incorporated intermittent fasting into her lifestyle under the supervision of her cardiologist. By following a 16/8 fasting schedule and making heart-healthy food choices on eating days, Linda achieved significant improvements in her cholesterol levels and cardiovascular health. Her story illustrates how intermittent fasting can be a valuable tool for heart health management.

Betty's Vibrant Aging at 76. Betty, at 76, was determined to age vibrantly. She embraced intermittent fasting as part of her comprehensive wellness plan. With guidance from a registered dietitian, she followed the 5:2 fasting method. Betty's journey resulted in increased energy, better sleep quality, and a stronger sense of vitality. Her story demonstrates how intermittent fasting can contribute to overall well-being and an active lifestyle in later years.

Ruth's Weight Management Success at 70. Ruth, at 70, was facing weight-related health concerns. She decided to explore intermittent fasting with guidance from her healthcare provider. Adopting a 14-hour daily fasting window, Ruth successfully managed her weight and saw improvements in her metabolic health. Her story highlights the potential of intermittent fasting as a sustainable approach to weight management for older women.

Chapter 2: Navigating the Aging Process

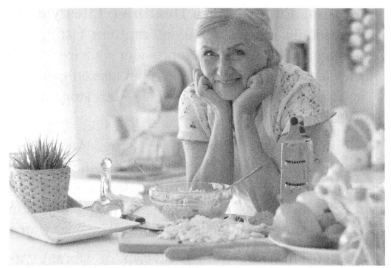

As women gracefully step into their seventies, they embark on a remarkable journey filled with wisdom, experiences, and the joys of life. However, this golden decade is also accompanied by unique physiological changes that can present certain challenges. Understanding these changes is the first step towards finding effective solutions, and intermittent fasting emerges as a promising strategy to address these challenges.

2.1 Physiological Changes Women Experience After 70 and How Fasting Can Address These Challenges

Metabolism: The Aging Catalyst. One of the most significant physiological changes women encounter after the age of 70 is a shift in metabolism. Metabolism tends to slow down, and the body may become less efficient at burning calories. This shift often leads to weight gain and increased fat accumulation, especially around the abdominal area. However, it's crucial to note that metabolism is not a fixed destiny. Intermittent fasting can play a pivotal role in reinvigorating metabolic function.

Hormonal Shifts: Navigating Hormone Fluctuations. Hormonal changes are a hallmark of the aging process. Post-menopause, women experience a decrease in estrogen levels, which can impact bone health, muscle mass, and overall vitality. These hormonal shifts may also influence appetite and the way the body stores fat. Intermittent fasting provides a valuable tool to navigate these hormone-related changes by promoting better hormone regulation and fat utilization.

Muscle Mass Maintenance: Overcoming Sarcopenia. Another challenge women face as they age is the loss of muscle mass, a condition known as sarcopenia. Reduced muscle mass can lead to decreased strength, mobility issues, and a higher risk of falls and fractures. Intermittent fasting, combined with adequate protein intake and strength training, can support muscle preservation and functional independence.

Digestive Changes: Enhancing Nutrient Absorption. Aging can bring about changes in digestion, including reduced stomach acid production and slower gastrointestinal motility. These changes can affect nutrient absorption and digestive comfort. Intermittent fasting, when practiced mindfully, can offer benefits like improved digestion, enhanced nutrient absorption, and reduced gastrointestinal discomfort.

Bone Health: Guarding Against Osteoporosis. Osteoporosis, a condition characterized by weakened bones, is a common concern for older women. Maintaining bone density is crucial to prevent fractures. While fasting doesn't directly impact bone health, it can contribute to weight management and improved metabolic function, both of which indirectly support bone health.

Inflammation and Cellular Health. Chronic inflammation and cellular damage are associated with aging and can contribute to various health issues. Intermittent fasting triggers a process called autophagy—a cellular "cleanup" mechanism that removes damaged cells and proteins. This promotes cellular repair and regeneration, potentially reducing the risk of age-related diseases and supporting longevity.

Cognitive Function. Cognitive health becomes increasingly significant with age. The fear of cognitive decline and conditions like Alzheimer's disease can be daunting. Intermittent fasting has shown promise in this regard. It stimulates the production of brain-derived neurotrophic factor (BDNF), a protein associated with brain health and the formation of new neurons. By promoting mental clarity and sharpness, intermittent fasting can help women maintain cognitive vitality well into their seventies and beyond.

Heart Health. Heart disease is a leading cause of concern for older adults. Intermittent fasting has been linked to improvements in heart health by reducing risk factors such as high blood pressure, cholesterol levels, and inflammation. Fasting periods can give the cardiovascular system a break and support overall heart function, contributing to a healthier and longer life.

Emotional Well-being. Aging often comes with emotional challenges, including feelings of isolation and depression. Intermittent fasting offers an opportunity for self-care and empowerment. It can boost self-esteem and provide a sense of accomplishment, which can positively impact emotional well-being. Additionally, fasting may stimulate the production of mood-enhancing neurotransmitters, helping to combat feelings of sadness or anxiety.

Vision and Eye Health. Vision changes are common as we age, and eye health is a significant concern for women over 70. Some age-related eye conditions can impact daily life, such as cataracts and macular degeneration. Intermittent fasting may support eye health by reducing oxidative stress and inflammation, factors that contribute to these conditions. Including antioxidant-rich foods in your diet during eating windows can further support your vision.

Sleep Quality. Maintaining restful sleep becomes crucial in later years. Poor sleep can exacerbate various health issues and reduce overall well-being. Intermittent fasting can positively influence sleep patterns by stabilizing blood sugar levels and promoting hormonal balance. A consistent fasting schedule can help regulate circadian rhythms, leading to better sleep quality and daytime alertness.

Social Engagement. Loneliness and social isolation can impact mental and emotional health in older women. Engaging in fasting as a lifestyle choice can foster a sense of community and connection. Joining online support groups or local communities of individuals practicing intermittent fasting can provide a sense of belonging and support, mitigating feelings of isolation.

Holistic Well-being. I am aware that I frequently insist on this topic. But embracing a holistic approach to well-being is essential in one's seventies. Intermittent fasting aligns with this philosophy, as it encourages mindful eating, self-awareness, and self-care. This approach extends beyond physical health, emphasizing emotional, mental, and spiritual well-being, fostering a sense of harmony in life.

2.2 Integrating Intermittent Fasting into Your Lifestyle and Building Confidence

As women enter their seventies, they often find themselves reflecting on their health and well-being. The years have brought with them a wealth of experiences, and the desire to enjoy the present and future to the fullest is paramount. It's at this juncture that many women consider embracing new approaches to health, and intermittent fasting emerges as a compelling option.

Integrating Intermittent Fasting into Your Lifestyle

Integrating intermittent fasting into your life is not just about following a trend or adopting a short-term diet. It's about making a conscious choice for a healthier future. While the concept of fasting may seem daunting, especially if it's new to you, remember that it's not a drastic or unsustainable approach. It's a lifestyle choice that you can adapt to your unique needs and preferences. One of the first steps in integrating intermittent fasting into your lifestyle is to start gradually. You don't need to dive into an advanced fasting schedule right away. Instead, consider a gentler approach, such as the 12/12 method, where you fast for 12 hours and eat during the remaining 12 hours of the day. This allows your body to adjust gradually to the fasting periods.

Building Confidence to Begin Your Journey

Building confidence to embark on your intermittent fasting journey is essential. Confidence comes not just from knowledge but also from experience and self-assurance. Here are some key strategies to help you build that confidence:

- ✓ **Education:** Take the time to learn about intermittent fasting. Understand its principles, benefits, and various methods. Knowledge is a powerful tool that dispels fear and uncertainty.

- ✓ **Start Slowly:** Begin with shorter fasting periods and gradually extend them as you become more comfortable. Starting with a 12-hour fast, as mentioned earlier, is an excellent way to ease into it.

- ✓ **Listen to Your Body:** Pay attention to how your body responds to fasting. Tune in to hunger cues and respect them. Remember, fasting should not lead to deprivation or excessive discomfort.

- ✓ **Seek Support:** Consider joining a community or support group of individuals who practice intermittent fasting. Sharing experiences and insights can boost your confidence and provide valuable guidance.

- ✓ **Set Realistic Goals:** Define your goals for intermittent fasting. Whether it's weight management, improved energy, or enhanced overall health, having clear objectives can keep you motivated.

- ✓ **Stay Flexible:** Intermittent fasting is not a one-size-fits-all approach. Be flexible and willing to adjust your fasting schedule to suit your lifestyle and preferences.

By taking these steps, you'll gradually integrate intermittent fasting into your daily routine and build the confidence needed to embark on this transformative journey. Remember that it's a process, and like any journey, it's about the experiences and discoveries along the way. As you move forward with confidence, you'll be better equipped to embrace the unique benefits of intermittent fasting for women over 70.

2.3 Dietary Options, Supplements, and Resources for Success

Exploring dietary options and supplements tailored to the unique needs of older women embarking on their intermittent fasting journey is an essential aspect of ensuring a successful and fulfilling experience. In addition, accessing valuable resources and tools to monitor your progress and maintain motivation will significantly contribute to your journey's long-term success.

Dietary Choices for Older Women Practicing Intermittent Fasting

As a woman over 70, it's crucial to focus on nutrient-dense foods that support your overall health and well-being. While intermittent fasting offers flexibility in when you eat, the quality of your meals remains paramount. Consider incorporating the following dietary strategies:

- ✓ **Whole Foods:** Prioritize whole, unprocessed foods rich in vitamins, minerals, and antioxidants. Opt for plenty of fruits, vegetables, lean proteins, and whole grains in your diet,

- ✓ **Protein Intake:** Adequate protein intake is essential for maintaining muscle mass and overall vitality. Include sources of lean protein like poultry, fish, beans, and legumes in your meals.

- ✓ **Healthy Fats:** Include sources of healthy fats, such as avocados, nuts, seeds, and olive oil, to support brain health and overall well-being.

- ✓ **Hydration:** Staying adequately hydrated is especially important as we age. Aim to drink plenty of water throughout the day to support digestion and overall health.

- ✓ **Supplements:** Consult with a healthcare professional or registered dietitian to determine if you have specific nutritional needs or deficiencies that require supplementation. Supplements like vitamin D and B12 may be beneficial for older adults.

Resources and Tools for Progress Tracking and Motivation

Maintaining motivation and tracking your progress are key factors in sustaining your intermittent fasting journey. Here are some valuable resources and tools to consider.

1. Fasting Apps

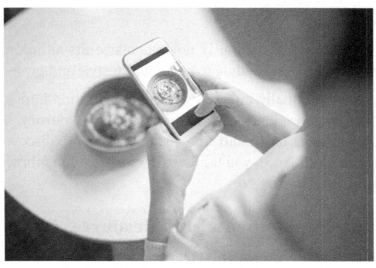

Several smartphone apps are designed to help you schedule and track your fasting windows, and many of them are user-friendly, making them accessible even with the help of family members or grandchildren. These apps can send reminders, record fasting hours, and provide insights into your fasting journey. Here are a few popular fasting apps that you can explore:

- ✓ **Zero - Fasting Tracker:** Zero is a straightforward fasting app that offers customizable fasting schedules and allows you to track your progress easily. It's known for its user-friendly interface, making it suitable for individuals of all ages.

- ✓ **Life Fasting Tracker:** Life offers a supportive community along with fasting tracking features. You can join groups, share your progress, and access resources to stay motivated.

- ✓ **MyFast:** MyFast provides a simple and intuitive platform for tracking your fasting hours. It's designed to be user-friendly and is a great choice for beginners.

- ✓ **FastHabit:** FastHabit allows you to create personalized fasting plans and offers visual tracking of your fasting progress. It's a handy tool for those looking for a flexible approach.

- ✓ **Vora - Fasting Tracker:** Vora is known for its clean and easy-to-navigate interface. It provides fasting tracking options and the ability to join fasting communities for support and inspiration.

These apps are readily available for download on most smartphone app stores, and you can explore their features to determine which one aligns best with your preferences and needs. Don't hesitate to seek assistance from family members or friends to help you get started with these apps. They can be valuable tools in your intermittent fasting journey.

2. Meal Planning

Create meal plans that align with your fasting schedule. Having a structured meal plan can make it easier to adhere to your chosen fasting method.

Do you have no idea how to do it? No worries!

Towards the end of this book, I've prepared something special for you. As you near the final chapters, you'll find a collection of recipes tailored for intermittent fasting, covering every meal of the day. These recipes are created with the nutritional needs and preferences of older women in mind. Also, I've developed a comprehensive 60-day meal plan that takes the guesswork out of meal planning. It will help you get started on your fasting journey with confidence, ensuring you enjoy balanced and satisfying meals. With these resources, you'll have all the tools you need to integrate intermittent fasting into your life seamlessly.

3. Support Groups

Joining a supportive community of individuals practicing intermittent fasting can be an incredibly valuable resource on your journey. These groups offer encouragement, advice, and a sense of camaraderie. You'll find various options to connect with like-minded individuals, both online and offline.

- ✓ **Online Forums and Social Media Groups:** The digital age has made it easier than ever to connect with people who share your interests. There are numerous online forums and social media groups dedicated to intermittent fasting. Websites like Reddit host vibrant communities where you can ask questions, share your experiences, and seek guidance. Facebook groups also provide a platform for joining discussions and finding local fasting buddies. Simply use your preferred search engine or social media platform to find relevant groups, and don't hesitate to ask your tech-savvy family members or grandchildren for assistance in navigating these online spaces.

- ✓ **Local Meetup Groups:** If you prefer face-to-face interactions, consider joining or starting a local intermittent fasting meetup group. Websites like Meetup.com can help you locate or create such groups in your area. Meeting in person allows you to form deeper connections, share meals, and offer and receive hands-on support. It's also an opportunity to learn from each other's experiences and potentially form lasting friendships.

4. Nutritionist or Dietitian

Consider consulting with a nutritionist or dietitian who specializes in intermittent fasting for personalized guidance and meal planning tailored to your specific needs.

5. Progress Journal

Maintaining a journal can be an invaluable tool for tracking your intermittent fasting journey. In your journal, you can record not only your experiences and challenges but also your remarkable successes along the way. This journal will become a source of motivation and reflection, allowing you to appreciate how far you've come. Moreover, it can provide valuable insights into your personal fasting patterns and preferences. As a special resource towards the end of this book, you'll find an Intermittent Fasting Tracker.

This tool is designed specifically for women over 70 embarking on their intermittent fasting journey. It will help you meticulously monitor your progress, keep tabs on your weight, and document your experiences as you practice intermittent fasting. With this tracker, you'll have a structured way to record your daily fasting periods, track your meals, and make informed adjustments to your fasting routine as needed. It will be your personal companion in this transformative journey.

2.4 How To Integrate Traditional Medicine And Natural Remedies With Intermittent Fasting

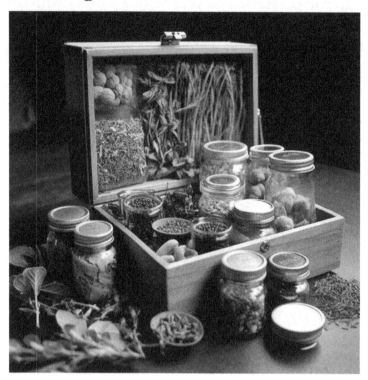

Integrating traditional medicine and natural remedies with intermittent fasting can provide a comprehensive approach to achieving optimal health and well-being, especially for women over 70. This synergy between ancient healing practices and modern dietary strategies offers a holistic approach that addresses the unique needs of older individuals.

Traditional Medicine and Herbal Remedies

Many traditional healing systems, such as Ayurveda, Traditional Chinese Medicine, and Native American herbalism, have relied on the use of medicinal herbs and natural remedies for centuries. These time-tested practices recognize the importance of balancing the body and mind for overall health. By integrating elements of traditional medicine into your intermittent fasting routine, you can tap into the wisdom of these ancient traditions. For example, herbal teas and infusions can support digestion, reduce inflammation, and promote relaxation. Ginger and peppermint teas can soothe the stomach during fasting periods, while chamomile and valerian root teas can aid in relaxation and sleep. Supplements derived from natural sources can complement your intermittent fasting journey.

Here are some natural remedies and supplements to consider:

- ✓ **Turmeric:** Known for its anti-inflammatory properties, turmeric may help reduce inflammation in the body, which can be beneficial for overall health.

- ✓ **Omega-3 Fatty Acids:** Omega-3 supplements, such as fish oil or flaxseed oil, can support heart health and cognitive function.

- ✓ **Probiotics:** Maintaining gut health is crucial, especially as we age. Probiotic supplements can promote a healthy gut microbiome.

- ✓ **Vitamin D:** Many older adults are deficient in vitamin D, which plays a vital role in bone health and immune function. A supplement may be necessary, especially for those with limited sun exposure.

- ✓ **Ashwagandha:** This adaptogenic herb may help reduce stress and support overall well-being. It has been used in Ayurvedic medicine for its calming and balancing effects.

- ✓ **Aloe Vera:** Known for its soothing properties, aloe vera can support digestive health and help alleviate occasional digestive discomfort.

- ✓ **Ginseng:** Ginseng, particularly Korean or Panax ginseng, is believed to boost energy, improve cognitive function, and enhance overall vitality.

- ✓ **Echinacea:** This herbal remedy is often used to support the immune system and reduce the severity and duration of colds and respiratory infections.

- ✓ **Magnesium:** Magnesium supplements can help support muscle and nerve function, bone health, and overall relaxation. Some older adults may have low magnesium levels.

- ✓ **Melatonin:** Melatonin supplements may aid in regulating sleep patterns, particularly for those experiencing sleep disturbances.

- ✓ **Hawthorn:** Hawthorn is used in traditional herbal medicine to support heart health and may help manage blood pressure within a healthy range.

- ✓ **Green Tea Extract:** Green tea contains antioxidants called catechins, which may support cellular health and metabolism.

- ✓ **Rhodiola Rosea:** This adaptogenic herb may help reduce fatigue, enhance mood, and improve overall mental and physical resilience.

- ✓ **Probiotics:** Probiotic supplements containing various strains of beneficial bacteria can support digestive and immune health.

- ✓ **Ginger:** Ginger is known for its anti-inflammatory and digestive properties. It can help alleviate stomach discomfort and aid digestion.

- ✓ **Berberine:** This plant extract has been linked to better blood sugar regulation and weight management.

- ✓ **Flaxseeds:** Flaxseeds are a source of dietary fiber and omega-3 fatty acids. They can help regulate bowel movements and promote heart health.

- ✓ **Chinese Magnolia:** Chinese magnolia bark extract has been used to reduce stress and promote mental calmness.
- ✓ **Black Pepper:** Black pepper contains piperine, which can enhance the absorption of certain nutrients, including curcumin.
- ✓ **Blueberries:** Blueberries are rich in antioxidants and can support eye health and cognitive function.
- ✓ **Peppermint Tea:** Peppermint tea is known for its digestive properties and can help reduce gastrointestinal discomfort.
- ✓ **Raisins:** Raisins are a natural snack option that can provide slow-release energy during fasting periods.

Integrating traditional medicine and natural remedies into your fasting routine should be done with guidance. Consult a healthcare provider, preferably one experienced in integrative medicine, to create a personalized plan. They can assess your specific health needs, recommend appropriate supplements or remedies, and ensure that they complement your intermittent fasting schedule. By combining the principles of traditional medicine and the benefits of natural remedies with intermittent fasting, you can create a comprehensive approach to health and wellness that addresses the unique concerns of women over 70. This integrated strategy prioritizes both physical and mental well-being, contributing to a balanced and vibrant life.

2.5 Special Considerations and Risks

Intermittent fasting is a powerful tool for improving health, but it's crucial to understand how it may affect women over 70 differently due to unique physiological factors and potential risks involved. Here, we'll explore these considerations and how to mitigate associated risks.

1. Nutrient Intake and Absorption. As we age, our bodies may have a reduced ability to absorb certain nutrients efficiently. When practicing intermittent fasting, it's essential to ensure that your meals are nutritionally dense. Incorporating a variety of colorful fruits and vegetables, lean proteins, and whole grains is key. Additionally, consider consulting with a healthcare provider or registered dietitian to address any specific nutrient concerns.

2. Medication Interactions. Many women over 70 are on medications to manage various health conditions. Intermittent fasting can potentially affect how medications are absorbed and metabolized. It's vital to consult with your healthcare provider before starting an intermittent fasting regimen, especially if you're taking prescription medications. They can offer guidance on medication timing and potential adjustments.

3. Dehydration. Fasting periods can increase the risk of dehydration, which can be particularly concerning for older adults. It's essential to stay adequately hydrated by drinking water during non-fasting hours. Herbal teas and hydration-rich foods like cucumbers and watermelon can also contribute to your fluid intake. Be attentive to signs of dehydration, such as dry mouth or dark urine, and take steps to prevent it.

4. Muscle Mass Preservation. Maintaining muscle mass is crucial for overall health, especially for women over 70. Intermittent fasting can help with weight management but may also result in muscle loss if not done correctly. To counteract this, include sufficient protein in your diet and engage in resistance or strength training exercises. Consult a fitness professional to create a safe and effective exercise plan that aligns with your fasting schedule.

5. Low Blood Sugar (Hypoglycemia)

Intermittent fasting can lead to drops in blood sugar levels, potentially causing symptoms like dizziness, fatigue, and confusion. This can be particularly risky for older adults. To prevent low blood sugar, opt for a gentler fasting approach and avoid overly extended fasting periods. If you experience symptoms of hypoglycemia, break your fast with a small, balanced meal.

6. Bone Health. Older women are at a higher risk of osteoporosis, and fasting could potentially impact bone health if calcium and vitamin D intake aren't adequate. Ensure you're including dairy products, leafy greens, and fortified foods in your diet. If you have concerns about bone health, consult with a healthcare provider for personalized recommendations.

7. Cognitive Health. Intermittent fasting has shown promise in supporting cognitive health, but it's vital to approach it cautiously. If you have any neurodegenerative conditions like dementia or Alzheimer's disease, consult with a healthcare provider before starting intermittent fasting. They can help tailor an approach that minimizes risks and maximizes potential benefits.

8. Metabolism and Hormonal Changes. Aging can bring about shifts in metabolism and hormonal balance. Women over 70 may experience changes in insulin sensitivity and hormonal fluctuations. Intermittent fasting can help regulate some of these factors but may also require close monitoring, especially if you have underlying health conditions. Working with a healthcare provider or nutritionist to manage hormonal changes and metabolic health is advisable.

9. Immune Function. A robust immune system becomes increasingly crucial with age. Intermittent fasting can enhance autophagy, a cellular process that eliminates damaged components and supports immune function. However, fasting should not compromise your immune system. Ensure that you're receiving adequate nutrients and consider immune-boosting foods like citrus fruits, berries, and immune-supportive supplements if necessary.

10. Individualized Approach. Every woman over 70 is unique, and what works well for one person may not be suitable for another. It's crucial to recognize that there's no one-size-fits-all approach to intermittent fasting. Incorporating intermittent fasting into your lifestyle as a woman over 70 can yield numerous health advantages, but it's essential to navigate it wisely. Consulting with healthcare professionals, staying informed, and monitoring your body's responses will help you embrace this approach safely and effectively.

Chapter 3: Exercise and Intermittent Fasting

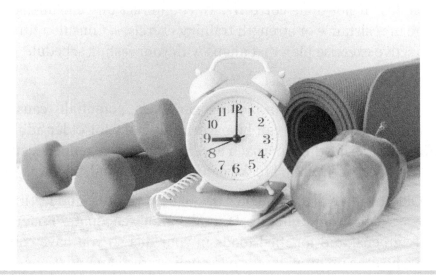

3.1 Synergy Between Intermittent Fasting and Physical Activity

Physical activity plays a pivotal role in our overall well-being, particularly as we age. When combined with intermittent fasting, it can create a powerful synergy that contributes to optimal aging. In this section, we will explore the unique benefits of incorporating exercise into your intermittent fasting routine and how it can positively impact women over 70.

Tailored Exercise for Optimal Aging

As we age, our bodies naturally undergo changes in muscle mass, bone density, and metabolism. To address these changes effectively, it's crucial to engage in exercise routines that are specifically tailored to the needs of women over 70. Here's what you need to know:

- ✓ **Strength Training:** Incorporating strength training exercises can help preserve and even increase muscle mass. This is particularly important for older adults as it can support mobility and independence.

- ✓ **Flexibility and Balance:** Gentle stretching exercises can enhance flexibility and balance, reducing the risk of falls and injuries. Activities like yoga or tai chi are excellent choices.

- ✓ **Aerobic Exercise:** Regular cardiovascular exercise, such as brisk walking or swimming, promotes heart health and stamina. It's vital for maintaining overall fitness.

- ✓ **Low-Impact Options:** Consider low-impact exercises to protect joints and reduce the risk of injury. Activities like cycling or water aerobics are gentle on the body.

Synergy with Intermittent Fasting

Intermittent fasting complements your exercise routine in several ways:

- ✓ **Fat Utilization:** During fasting periods, your body becomes more efficient at using stored fat for energy. This can enhance your endurance during workouts and promote weight management.

- ✓ **Muscle Preservation:** Intermittent fasting encourages the preservation of lean muscle mass, even during weight loss. This is crucial for maintaining strength and mobility.

- ✓ **Improved Recovery:** Fasting may promote cellular repair and recovery processes. This can lead to reduced post-workout soreness and faster healing of exercise-related injuries.

- ✓ **Enhanced Mental Clarity:** Intermittent fasting can improve cognitive function, which can enhance your focus and motivation for regular exercise.

Finding the Right Balance

It's essential to strike a balance between intermittent fasting and exercise. Listen to your body and adjust your fasting schedule to accommodate your workout routine. Here are some tips:

- Consider fasting during the non-exercising hours of your day to ensure you have the necessary energy for your workouts.

- Stay hydrated during fasting periods, especially before and after exercise.

- Pay attention to how your body responds to fasting and exercise. If you feel lightheaded, weak, or overly fatigued, it might be an indicator to adjust your fasting window or eat a small, balanced meal before working out.

In summary, exercise and intermittent fasting can be powerful allies in your journey to optimal aging. Tailoring your workout routine to your specific needs as a woman over 70 and finding the right balance between fasting and exercise can result in improved overall health, vitality, and quality of life.

3.2 Holistic Wellness Practices for Optimal Aging

As I have already said before, in the pursuit of optimal aging, it's essential to look beyond just diet and exercise. Holistic wellness practices, such as yoga and mindfulness, play a significant role in supporting your mental and physical health as a woman over 70.

The Power of Yoga. Yoga offers a versatile range of practices suitable for various fitness levels. As a woman over 70, you can find yoga routines that are gentle, low-impact, and designed to enhance flexibility, balance, and strength. These practices are tailored to your unique requirements, making them accessible and enjoyable. Yoga can bring about physical benefits by improving joint flexibility, alleviating stiffness, and enhancing posture. It's an excellent way to maintain or regain mobility, which can be especially valuable as we age. Moreover, yoga can help manage chronic conditions like arthritis and lower back pain. Beyond its physical aspects, yoga incorporates mindfulness and deep breathing. These aspects of yoga can reduce stress, promote relaxation, and improve sleep quality—essential components of holistic well-being. Yoga's meditative qualities can enhance your mental clarity and emotional resilience, contributing to a more balanced and peaceful state of mind.

Mindfulness for a Balanced Life. Mindfulness practices involve staying present in the moment without judgment. This can be particularly beneficial for women over 70 who may face various life changes and stressors. Mindfulness techniques can help you manage stress, anxiety, and feelings of overwhelm more effectively.

By cultivating mindfulness, you can develop a deeper understanding of your emotions and thought patterns. This self-awareness allows you to respond to life's challenges with greater emotional balance and resilience. Additionally, mindfulness practices have been shown to enhance cognitive function, including memory and focus. This can support your mental acuity and overall brain health as you age.

Holistic Wellness as a Lifestyle. Embracing holistic wellness practices isn't about quick fixes or temporary solutions. It's a lifestyle choice that nurtures your mental and physical health over the long term. As you incorporate yoga and mindfulness into your routine, you're not only addressing physical concerns but also nurturing your emotional and mental well-being.. Remember, it's never too late to start. These practices can be integrated into your daily life, offering you the opportunity to live your later years with vitality and fulfillment.

3.3 30-Day Exercise Plan Designed For Women Over 70

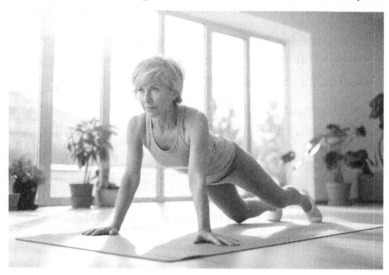

Here is a 30-day exercise plan designed for seniors, specifically tailored for women over 70 looking to integrate exercise with intermittent fasting. This plan is designed to be gentle and progressive, promoting increased mobility, strength, and flexibility, all while being mindful of the needs of women over 70. It complements the intermittent fasting approach, contributing to an overall healthy and vital lifestyle. Remember to listen to your body and adjust the plan as needed to suit your individual comfort level and capabilities.

Week 1-2: Building a Foundation

Day 1: Gentle Morning Stretching Routine (10 minutes)

- Start with a seated position on a comfortable chair.

- Gently stretch your arms overhead and reach towards the ceiling while taking a deep breath.

- Slowly twist your upper body to the left and right, holding each stretch for a few seconds.

- Extend your legs and point and flex your toes.

- Perform neck stretches by gently tilting your head from side to side.
- Finish with deep breathing exercises, inhaling and exhaling slowly.

Day 2: Rest or Light Walking (15-20 minutes)

- Choose a safe and flat walking surface.
- Wear comfortable shoes with proper arch support.
- Walk at a comfortable pace, focusing on good posture and taking steady, deep breaths.

Day 3: Chair Yoga for Beginners (15-20 minutes)

- Begin in a seated position with your feet flat on the floor.
- Follow along with a chair yoga video or instructor.
- Chair yoga typically includes gentle stretches, seated poses, and controlled breathing exercises.

Day 4: Rest or Light Walking (15-20 minutes)

Day 5: Seated Leg Lifts (2 sets of 10 reps per leg)

- Sit on a sturdy chair with your back straight and feet flat on the floor.
- Hold onto the sides of the chair for balance.
- Lift one leg straight out in front of you while keeping the knee slightly bent.
- Lower the leg back down and repeat for the desired number of reps.
- Switch to the other leg.

Day 6: Rest or Light Walking (15-20 minutes)

Day 7: Gentle Morning Stretching Routine (10 minutes)

CONTINUE WITH THE SAME SCHEDULE FOR WEEK 2!

Week 3-4: Progressing and Enhancing Mobility

Day 1: Seated Marching (2 sets of 20 reps)

- Sit on a sturdy chair with your back straight and feet flat on the floor.
- Hold onto the sides of the chair for balance.
- March in place by lifting one knee toward your chest and then lowering it.
- Repeat for the desired number of reps, alternating legs.

Day 2: Rest or Light Walking (15-20 minutes)

Day 3: Chair Yoga for Flexibility (20 minutes)

Day 4: Rest or Light Walking (15-20 minutes)

Day 5: Seated Arm Raises (2 sets of 10 reps per arm)

- Sit on a sturdy chair with your back straight and feet flat on the floor.

- Hold a lightweight object (like a water bottle) in one hand.

- Slowly raise your arm with the object straight up in front of you.

- Lower the arm back down and repeat for the desired number of reps.

- Switch to the other arm.

Day 6: Rest or Light Walking (15-20 minutes)

Day 7: Gentle Morning Stretching Routine (10 minutes)

CONTINUE WITH THE SAME SCHEDULE FOR WEEK 4!

On Day 30, you can choose to revisit your favorite exercises or activities from the past 30 days. This is a day to celebrate your achievements and the progress you've made on your fitness journey!

Tips:

- ✓ Perform each exercise slowly and deliberately, focusing on proper form and breathing. Stay hydrated throughout your exercise routine.

- ✓ If you experience any discomfort or pain, stop immediately and consult with a healthcare professional.

- ✓ It's essential to maintain a balanced diet during intermittent fasting, ensuring you receive the necessary nutrients to support your exercise regimen.

- ✓ Prioritize rest and recovery days to allow your body to adapt and prevent overexertion.

Chapter 4: Beyond the Book: Resources and Community

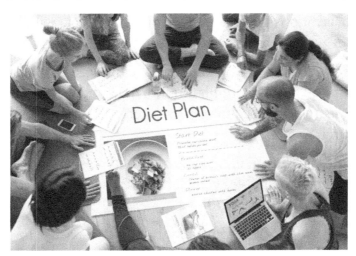

4.1 Discovering Reliable Resources: Reputable Websites

Intermittent fasting is a field of health and wellness that's continually evolving, with researchers discovering new insights into its potential benefits, especially for women over 70. However, before delving into the world of intermittent fasting research, it's essential to distinguish credible sources from the less reputable ones. In an age of abundant information, not all sources are created equal.

There are several reputable websites and online platforms where you can find well-curated information about intermittent fasting and its benefits for older women. Some examples include websites run by renowned medical institutions, universities, and reputable health organizations, such as:

- ✓ **Mayo Clinic:** The Mayo Clinic's website offers comprehensive and well-researched articles on health and wellness topics, including intermittent fasting for older women. Their content is authored by medical experts and is known for its reliability and accuracy.

- ✓ **Harvard Health Publishing:** Harvard Medical School's health publishing arm provides valuable insights into various health topics, including intermittent fasting. Their articles are evidence-based and reviewed by medical professionals.

- ✓ **National Institute on Aging (NIA):** NIA, a part of the National Institutes of Health (NIH), is dedicated to research on aging-related issues. Their website is a trusted source for information on aging, health, and lifestyle, making it an excellent resource for women over 70 interested in intermittent fasting.

4.2 Discovering Reliable Resources: Academic Journals

Peer-reviewed academic journals are a valuable resource for in-depth scientific research on intermittent fasting. Navigating these journals may seem daunting, but I will try to guide you on how to access them and effectively interpret research papers. This will empower you to stay informed about the latest findings and understand their implications for your health.

Accessing Academic Journals:

- ✓ **University Libraries:** Many universities offer public access to their libraries, which often include subscriptions to academic journals. Check with your local university or library to see if they provide free or low-cost access.

- ✓ **Online Databases:** Several online platforms grant access to academic journals for a fee or with a subscription. Some popular options include JSTOR, PubMed, and Google Scholar. You can search for specific topics, such as "intermittent fasting and aging," to find relevant research papers.

- ✓ **ResearchGate:** ResearchGate is a platform where researchers share their work. While not all papers are freely accessible, you can request copies directly from the authors, and they may be willing to share their findings.

- ✓ **Open Access Journals:** Some journals provide free access to their articles, making it easier for the public to read and benefit from scientific research. Look for journals with open-access options in your areas of interest.

Deciphering Research Papers

- ✓ **Abstract:** Start by reading the abstract, a summary of the research paper's key findings and purpose. This will help you determine if the paper is relevant to your interests.

- ✓ **Introduction:** The introduction sets the stage for the study, explaining its background and objectives. It's a good section to understand the context and goals of the research.

- ✓ **Methods:** Pay attention to the methods section, which outlines how the study was conducted. Understanding the methodology is essential to assess the quality of the research.

- ✓ **Results:** Examine the results section for the main findings. Researchers typically present their data through tables, graphs, or charts. Try to grasp the core outcomes of the study.

- ✓ **Discussion:** In the discussion section, researchers interpret their findings and often highlight their implications. This is where you can gain insights into how the research relates to intermittent fasting and its effects on older women.

- ✓ **Conclusion:** Read the conclusion to get a concise summary of the study's main points and outcomes.

Reputable Academic Journals:

Here are some reputable academic journals known for their contributions to the field of nutrition and aging:

- ✓ **The Journals of Gerontology, Series A: Biological Sciences and Medical Sciences**

- ✓ **Aging Cell**

- ✓ **Nutrition and Aging**

- ✓ **The American Journal of Clinical Nutrition**

✓ **The Journals of Gerontology, Series B: Psychological Sciences and Social Sciences**

4.3 Connecting with Like-Minded Individuals

Your intermittent fasting journey can be more enjoyable and motivating when shared with a supportive community.

1. Online Forums

Online forums dedicated to intermittent fasting can be valuable hubs for sharing experiences, gaining knowledge, and seeking support from a like-minded community. Whether you have questions, want to share your progress, or simply connect with others on a similar journey, these forums provide a space to engage in discussions related to fasting. It's a great way to learn from others, share your challenges and successes, and stay motivated throughout your intermittent fasting journey. Here are some online forums that cater to individuals interested in intermittent fasting:

✓ **The Fasting Method Community:** This forum is hosted by Dr. Jason Fung's team and offers a supportive community of individuals practicing various forms of fasting. You can find discussions on fasting protocols, meal planning, and success stories.

✓ **Reddit's r/intermittentfasting:** Reddit hosts a thriving community of intermittent fasters who discuss their fasting routines, share tips, and provide motivation. It's a great place to ask questions and connect with people from around the world.

✓ **MyFitnessPal Forums:** MyFitnessPal, a popular fitness and nutrition app, has forums dedicated to intermittent fasting. You can join discussions on fasting, meal tracking, and health goals.

✓ **Bodybuilding.com Intermittent Fasting Forum:** If you're interested in combining intermittent fasting with fitness and bodybuilding, this forum offers insights into how fasting can complement an active lifestyle.

✓ **The 5:2 Diet Forum:** This forum focuses specifically on the 5:2 diet, a form of intermittent fasting. It's a resource for those following this particular fasting approach.

✓ **Facebook Groups:** Many Facebook groups are dedicated to intermittent fasting. Some groups are general, while others cater to specific fasting methods or demographics. You can search for groups that align with your interests and preferences.

2. Social Media Groups

Here are some recommendations for social media groups that are particularly welcoming and cater to the needs of older women:

✓ **Intermittent Fasting for Women Over 70 (Facebook Group):** This group is exclusively dedicated to older women who are exploring or practicing intermittent fasting. It offers a safe and supportive space to discuss topics related to fasting, share personal experiences, and seek advice from peers in the same age group.

- ✓ **Reddit's r/IF_People (Intermittent Fasting for People):** While not age-specific, this Reddit community is known for its inclusivity and respectful atmosphere. It's a place where individuals of all ages, including older women, discuss their intermittent fasting journeys, share success stories, and offer guidance.

- ✓ **The 16/8 Intermittent Fasting Group (Facebook Group):** If you're interested in the 16/8 fasting method, this group focuses on that specific approach. It's a platform for individuals to exchange tips, meal ideas, and encouragement related to the 16/8 method.

- ✓ **Fasting Over 60 (Facebook Group):** While not exclusively for women, this Facebook group caters to individuals over the age of 60 who are practicing intermittent fasting. It's a community where older adults can discuss their unique fasting experiences and support one another.

- ✓ **Women's Health and Fasting (Reddit's r/WomensHealth):** This subreddit covers a wide range of women's health topics, including intermittent fasting. It's a place to seek advice, engage in discussions, and learn from others about fasting and overall well-being.

- ✓ **Facebook Support Groups for Specific Fasting Methods:** Depending on your chosen fasting method, you can find Facebook support groups dedicated to that approach. For instance, if you're interested in the 5:2 diet, search for relevant groups where you can connect with like-minded individuals.

3. Local Meetup Groups

Local meetup groups can be an excellent way to establish in-person connections with like-minded individuals in your community who share an interest in intermittent fasting. While the availability of such groups can vary based on your location, here are some suggestions on how to find or start local meetup groups:

- ✓ **Meetup.com:** Meetup is a popular online platform that facilitates the creation of local groups centered around various interests, including health and wellness. You can visit Meetup.com and search for intermittent fasting or related keywords to find existing groups in your area. If you don't find one, consider starting your own meetup group tailored to older women interested in intermittent fasting.

- ✓ **Facebook Events:** Facebook often features local events and gatherings, including health and fitness-related meetups. Use Facebook's event search function to look for intermittent fasting meetups or wellness gatherings in your vicinity.

- ✓ **Community Centers and Gyms:** Contact local community centers, gyms, or wellness centers to inquire about any intermittent fasting or nutrition-related workshops, classes, or meetups they might be hosting.

- ✓ **Senior Centers:** If you're specifically interested in connecting with other older women, your local senior center might be a great place to start. Inquire about any wellness programs or nutrition discussions that align with your interests.

- ✓ **Online Forums:** Some online forums, such as those mentioned earlier, may have sections dedicated to organizing local meetups. Check these forums for announcements of local gatherings or consider posting a request to start one in your area.

- ✓ **Word of Mouth:** Don't underestimate the power of word of mouth. Mention your interest in intermittent fasting to friends, family, or acquaintances in your community. They might know of local groups or be interested in joining you to start one.

4.4 Involving Loved Ones

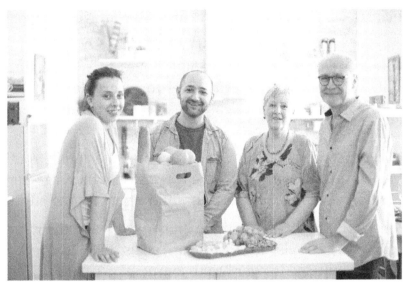

Support from family and friends is invaluable on your health journey. In this section, we'll discuss ways to involve your loved ones in your intermittent fasting endeavors. This can foster a positive atmosphere where your goals are understood, respected, and even adopted by those close to you. Here are some strategies for involving your family and enjoying the benefits together:

- ✓ **Family Meetings:** Schedule a family meeting to discuss your decision to try intermittent fasting. Explain the reasons behind your choice, emphasizing health benefits and personal goals. Encourage open dialogue, allowing each family member to express their thoughts and concerns.

- ✓ **Education for All:** Share educational resources about intermittent fasting with your family. Consider watching documentaries or reading books together that explain the science and potential advantages. This shared knowledge can foster understanding and unity.

- ✓ **Meal Planning as a Team:** Involve your family in meal planning. Collaborate on creating balanced and nutritious meals that align with your fasting schedule. This ensures that everyone's dietary needs are met while supporting your fasting goals.

- ✓ **Cooking Together:** Cooking can be a fun and bonding activity. Encourage family members to participate in meal preparation. This not only eases your workload but also allows everyone to be more mindful of ingredients and portion sizes.

✓ **Family Fasting Days:** Designate certain days or meals when the whole family practices intermittent fasting together. This shared experience can promote a sense of togetherness and commitment to a healthier lifestyle.

✓ **Supportive Environment:** Ensure that your family understands the importance of creating a supportive environment. This means refraining from eating tempting foods in front of you during your fasting window and offering words of encouragement.

✓ **Respect Individual Choices:** While you may be enthusiastic about intermittent fasting, it's essential to respect the choices of other family members. Not everyone may want to participate, and that's perfectly fine. Encourage autonomy in their dietary decisions.

✓ **Celebrate Milestones:** As you achieve milestones in your fasting journey, celebrate them as a family. Whether it's a special meal to break a longer fast or acknowledging improved health markers, shared celebrations reinforce your collective commitment to well-being.

✓ **Family Activity:** Incorporate physical activity into your family routine. Consider going for walks together, practicing yoga, or engaging in other age-appropriate exercises. Staying active as a family complements your intermittent fasting efforts.

✓ **Monitor Progress:** Encourage family members to track their progress, whether it's related to weight, energy levels, or other health goals. Regular check-ins can help you all stay motivated and connected in your health journeys.

4.5 Enlisting Supportive Friends: Encouraging Friends to Join Your Fasting Journey

Fasting doesn't have to be a solitary endeavor; it can be a shared experience with friends who can provide valuable support and motivation. Here are some ways to engage your friends in your intermittent fasting journey:

✓ **Educate Your Friends:** Share your knowledge about intermittent fasting with your friends. Explain the health benefits, the science behind it, and your personal reasons for embracing this lifestyle. Be open to addressing their questions and concerns.

✓ **Lead by Example:** Showcase your commitment to fasting through your own actions and results. As your friends witness the positive changes in your health and well-being, they may become more interested in joining you.

✓ **Plan Social Activities:** When arranging social gatherings, consider planning activities that align with your fasting schedule. Opt for non-food-centered outings like walks in the park, attending fitness classes, or engaging in hobbies that don't involve eating. This way, you can still enjoy quality time with your friends without the focus on food.

✓ **Share Recipes:** If you discover delicious and nutritious recipes that are suitable for intermittent fasting, don't hesitate to share them with your friends. Encourage them to try these recipes and discuss the benefits of incorporating them into their own diets.

- ✓ **Host Fasting Challenges:** Organize intermittent fasting challenges with your friends. Set specific goals, such as fasting for a certain number of hours or days, and track progress together. Friendly competition can be a great motivator.

- ✓ **Join Online Fasting Groups:** Explore online forums and social media groups related to intermittent fasting and invite your friends to join you. These platforms offer a sense of community and can provide additional support and advice.

- ✓ **Cook or Meal Prep Together:** Invite friends over for a meal preparation session. Prepare fasting-friendly meals together, share cooking tips, and enjoy a shared meal that aligns with your fasting schedules.

- ✓ **Celebrate Milestones:** When you or your friends reach fasting milestones or achieve health goals, celebrate these achievements together. Acknowledging progress reinforces your commitment to well-being.

- ✓ **Encourage Flexibility:** Be understanding of your friends' choices and preferences. Not everyone may be ready to embrace intermittent fasting, and that's okay. Encourage them to explore it at their own pace and offer support regardless of their decisions.

- ✓ **Be a Source of Support:** Just as you seek support from your friends, be a source of encouragement for them as well. Offer a listening ear, share your experiences, and celebrate their successes along the way.

Chapter 4: Breakfast Recipes For Intermittent Fasting

1. Chocolate Banana Smoothie

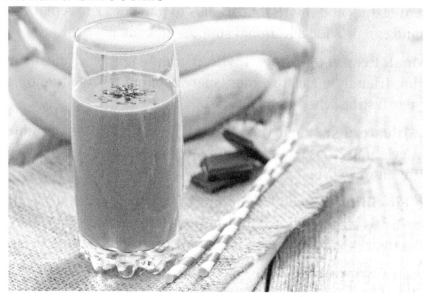

(Ready in: 5 minutes | Cook Duration: None | Persons: 2)

Necessary Items:

- Bananas, ripe and ready: 2
- Unsweetened cocoa powder: 2 tablespoons
- Milk, low-fat, or an almond variant for a non-dairy alternative: 1 cup
- Greek yogurt: 1/2 cup
- Honey or perhaps maple syrup (optional, to enhance sweetness): 1 tablespoon
- Vanilla extract: 1/2 teaspoon
- Ice cubes (optional, to adjust consistency): 1 cup

How to Prepare:

✓ Prepare the Ingredients: Peel and slice the ripe bananas.

✓ When all the ingredients are ready for preparation, all you have to do is take the bananas, cocoa, milk, Greek yogurt, honey, and vanilla extract, put them in the blender and combine.

✓ Add Ice Cubes: If you prefer a thicker smoothie, add a cup of ice cubes to the blender.

✓ The mixture must be made homogeneous and well blended. If it becomes too thick, you can add a little more milk.

✓ Taste and adjust the sweetness. If necessary, you can add more honey or maple syrup.

✓ Serve: Pour the chocolate banana smoothie into glasses and serve immediately.

Nutritional Info (per serving, without optional honey/maple syrup and ice cubes):
Calories: 175 kcal, Protein: 8g, Carbohydrates: 32g, Fat: 28g, Saturated Fat: 1g, Cholesterol: 8mg, Sodium: 64mg, Potassium: 627mg, Sugars: 16g

2. Spinach and Mushroom Omelette

(Ready in: 10 minutes | Cook Duration: 10 minutes | Persons: 2)

Necessary Items:

- Eggs, large and fresh: 4
- Spinach leaves, freshly washed and neatly chopped: 1 cup
- Mushrooms, sliced to a thin consistency: 1/2 cup
- Onion, finely diced: 1/4 cup
- Red bell pepper, chopped with precision: 1/4 cup
- Cheese, shredded (pick your preference, maybe cheddar or Swiss): 1/4 cup
- Season with salt and pepper as per your liking
- Olive oil or perhaps cooking spray: 2 teaspoons

How to Prepare:

- ✓ Egg Magic: Crack those eggs open, give them a good whisk, and introduce them to a pinch of salt and pepper. Let them mingle while you focus on the veggies.
- ✓ Veggie Prep: Give a fine chop to the spinach, mushrooms, onion, and vibrant red bell pepper.
- ✓ Vegetable Waltz: Get that skillet nice and warm with some olive oil dancing over medium-high heat. Invite the onion and red bell pepper to the party, letting them groove until they're just soft, which should be around 2 minutes.
- ✓ Mushroom Magic: Now, it's time for the mushrooms to join in. Let them sway and sizzle for about 3-4 minutes. You'll know it's time to move on when they're tender and have shared all their juicy secrets.
- ✓ Spinach Soirée: Toss in that spinach and watch as it gracefully wilts in just about 2 minutes.
- ✓ Egg Embrace: Cascade those whisked eggs over the dancing vegetables, ensuring everyone's bathed in that eggy goodness.
- ✓ Omelette Onstage: Dim the heat to a cozy medium-low and drape the skillet with a lid. Let the omelette perform alone for about 5 minutes or until it's got a firm grip on its edges.
- ✓ Cheesy Finale: With a flourish, sprinkle the shredded cheese on one side of the omelette, setting the stage for the grand finale.
- ✓ Encore: Gently persuade one side of the omelette to embrace the cheesy side with the help of a spatula. Let them harmonize for another 2 minutes until the cheese sings in melted joy and the omelette reaches perfection.
- ✓ Applause & Enjoy: Elegantly slide your culinary masterpiece onto a plate. Slice it down the middle, share the encore with another (or just double the treat for yourself), and savor it while it's still warm.

Nutritional Info: Calories: 230 kcal, Protein: 15g, Carbohydrates: 6g, Dietary Fiber: 2g, Sugars: 2g, Fat: 16g, Saturated Fat: 5g, Cholesterol: 389mg, Sodium: 367mg, Potassium: 438mg

3. Smoked Salmon Bagel

(Ready in: 5 minutes | Cook Duration: N/A | Persons: 2)

Necessary Items:

- Bagels, whole-grain, toasted after slicing: 2
- Smoked salmon, approximately 115g or 4 oz
- Cream cheese, low-fat variant, weighing around 115g or 4 oz
- Red onion, sliced with finesse: 1/4
- Capers: 2 tablespoons
- Dill sprigs, fresh, for that added touch
- Lemon wedges, to complement the serving

How to Prepare:

- ✓ Bagel Beginnings: Grab those hearty whole-grain bagels and slice them with flair, letting them bask in the toaster until they reach your ideal shade of golden brown.
- ✓ Creamy Canvass: Once they've had their toasty tan, lay out your bagel base and swath it generously with a luscious spread of low-fat cream cheese.
- ✓ Salmon Symphony: On this creamy foundation, drape delicate slices of that smoky salmon, letting it settle in luxuriously.
- ✓ Onion Overtones: Now, add some pizzazz with wafer-thin slices of red onion, ensuring they lay in perfect harmony atop the salmon.
- ✓ Caper Confetti: For a dash of oceanic surprise, scatter a handful of capers, letting them nestle amidst the onions.
- ✓ Dill Drama: Seal the ensemble with a dashing sprig of fresh dill, waving fragrantly above its delectable companions.
- ✓ Bagel Ballet's Finale: Crown your creation by placing the bagel's top half over the artfully assembled ingredients. For those who desire a citrusy crescendo, serve with lemon wedges waiting in the wings. Dive in and enjoy your flavor dance!

Nutritional Info: Calories: 340 kcal, Protein: 20g, Carbohydrates: 39g, Dietary Fiber: 5g, Sugars: 5g, Fat: 11g, Saturated Fat: 4g, Cholesterol: 32mg, Sodium: 620mg, Potassium: 225mg

4. Veggie Breakfast Burrito

(Ready in: 15 minutes | Cook Duration: 10 minutes | Persons: 2)

Necessary Items:

- Eggs, large and ready: 4
- Tortillas, whole-grain: 2
- Red bell pepper, chopped into small pieces: 1/2
- Green bell pepper, similarly diced: 1/2
- Onion, finely diced: 1/2
- Tomato, small and diced: 1
- Spinach leaves, baby variety: 1/2 cup
- Cheddar cheese, reduced-fat and shredded: 1/2 cup
- Olive oil: 1/2 teaspoon
- Season as per your preference with salt and pepper
- Sauce, if you fancy, for an enhanced serving experience.

How to Prepare:

- ✓ Veggie Prelude: In the realm of the skillet, let olive oil dance under medium fuel.

- ✓ Introduce the troupes: diced onions and the red and green bell pepper duo. Let them cook for a spell, around 3-4 minutes, until they're soft and their performance peaks.
- ✓ Egg Extravaganza: In your trusty mixing bowl, whip those eggs into a frothy frenzy. Release them onto the skillet, joining the veggie ensemble. Guide their dance, scrambling and twirling, until they're perfectly cooked, yet retaining a hint of dewy moisture.
- ✓ Spinach & Tomato Tango: Dim the fuel with a low heat setting and invite the tender baby spinach and vibrant diced tomato to join the act. As they dance, the spinach will gracefully wilt and the tomato will exude a touch of its juicy essence. A pinch of salt and pepper orchestrate the finishing notes.
- ✓ Burrito Ballad: Warm slightly your whole-grain tortillas, either with a gentle microwave hum or a griddle's heat. Lay them out, ready for their main act, bestowing upon each the mesmerizing egg and veggie concoction. To elevate the act, rain down a shower of shredded cheddar magic.
- ✓ The Great Roll-Up: Fold the tortilla's flanks inward, then choreograph its roll from its base, wrapping its treasures securely within.
- ✓ Curtain Call: Present your Veggie Breakfast Burrito masterpieces to an eager audience. For an encore, a side of spirited salsa awaits, amplifying each bite's spectacle.

Nutritional Info: Calories: 320 kcal, Protein: 18g, Carbohydrates: 24g, Dietary Fiber: 6g, Sugars: 4g, Fat: 17g, Saturated Fat: 5g, Cholesterol: 383mg, Sodium: 460mg, Potassium: 430mg

5. Ricotta Stuffed Crepes

(Ready in: 15 minutes | Cook Duration: 20 minutes | Persons: 2)

Necessary Items:

For the Crepes:

- All-purpose flour: 1 cup
- Eggs, large and fresh: 2
- Milk: 1 1/2 cups
- Sugar, granulated: 1 tablespoon
- Salt: 1/4 teaspoon
- Butter, unsalted and in liquid form: 2 tablespoons

For the Inner Delight:

- Ricotta cheese: 1 cup
- Sugar, powdered: 1/4 cup
- Vanilla extract: 1/2 teaspoon
- Lemon, just the zest: 1

For the Final Touch:

- Berries, fresh (consider strawberries, blueberries, or raspberries)
- Honey or perhaps maple syrup (only if you wish)
- Sugar, powdered, for a gentle sprinkle (completely optional)

How to Prepare:

- ✓ Crafting the Crepe Concoction: In your trusty blender, mix the esteemed all-purpose flour, the gallant eggs, the lush milk, the delightful sugar, and a hint of salt. Swirl them in harmony, and after a spell, fold in the liquid gold (melted butter) until it becomes a unified blend. Grant this mixture some peace, allowing it to stand for fifteen tranquil minutes.

- ✓ Crepe Cavalcade: Set your slick pan or crepe maker to a moderate flame. Bless it with a touch of butter. Drizzle in a scoop of your crafted concoction, ensuring it dances across, covering every nook and cranny. Allow it to bask for a minute or two until it starts radiating a golden hue. With confidence, turn the crepe to its other side and let it bask a little more.
- ✓ Ricotta Revelry: In a pristine bowl, conjure a silken ricotta blend sprinkled with powdered sugar, a hint of vanilla aura, and the zesty embrace of one lemon. Stir this ensemble until velvety.
- ✓ Crepes in Concert: Lay out your crepes and lavish them with the splendid ricotta concoction on one half, then tenderly fold to encapsulate the richness within.
- ✓ Final Flourish: Proudly display your ricotta-laden crepes adorned with jubilant berries. For the true connoisseurs, drizzle with nature's nectar-like honey or maple syrup or perhaps a gentle flurry of powdered sugar.

Nutritional Info: Calories: 375 kcal, Protein: 15g, Carbohydrates: 44g, Dietary Fiber: 1g, Sugars: 10g, Fat: 15g, Saturated Fat: 9g, Cholesterol: 144mg, Sodium: 243mg, Potassium: 216mg

6. Potato Hash

(Ready in: 15 minutes | Cook Duration: 25 minutes | Persons: 2)

Necessary Items:

- Potatoes, medium-sized, peeled and cubed: 2
- Onion, medium and finely diced: 1/2
- Bell pepper, color of your choice, chopped: 1
- Garlic, finely minced: 2 cloves
- Olive oil: 2 tablespoons

- Paprika: 1/2 teaspoon
- Thyme, dried: 1/2 teaspoon
- Season as per your preference with salt and black pepper
- Fresh parsley, chopped (a delightful optional garnish)

How to Prepare:

- ✓ Spud Prelude: Initiate the process by immersing the potato cubes into a pot of bubbling water. Allow them to simmer for roughly 5 minutes, achieving a tenderness that isn't quite complete. Once done, drain these half-cooked jewels and set them to rest.
- ✓ Golden Onion Elegy: In a pan, warm the olive essence under medium-high flame. Welcome the onions and garlic to this heated dance. Continue their sautéing ballet for about 2-3 minutes until the onions are put on a very tender.
- ✓ Potato-Pepper Promenade: Usher in the semi-tender potatoes and the vibrant bell pepper ribbons to the ensemble. Allow them to cook, rarely intervening, so they achieve a golden allure. Stir occasionally to guarantee a consistent gold-kissed hue.
- ✓ Spice Symphony: Sprint the pan's contents with sprinkles of paprika, whispers of dried thyme, a hint of salt, and a dash of black pepper. Mix them harmoniously, ensuring each morsel gets its fair share of this spicy melody. Continue the sizzling cook for about 10-15 minutes until the potatoes wear a golden, crisp robe.
- ✓ Final Flair: Upon completion of the opus, remove it from the flame's embrace. For those seeking an aesthetic encore, color with freshly-snipped parsley, lending a verdant pop.

✓ Plating Prologue: Offer up the Potato Hash as a morning's gastronomic delight. Revel in the heartwarming symphony of tastes with each morsel!

Nutritional Info: Calories: 273 kcal, Protein: 3g, Carbohydrates: 38g, Dietary Fiber: 5g, Sugars: 4g, Fat: 13g, Saturated Fat: 2g, Cholesterol: 0mg, Sodium: 28mg, Potassium: 727mg

---

7. Chickpea Scramble

(Ready in: 10 minutes ! Cook Duration: 15 minutes | Persons: 2)

Necessary Items:

- Chickpeas, from a 15 oz can, drained and given a rinse: 1 can
- Onion, medium in size and finely diced: 1/2
- Bell pepper, color of your choosing, chopped: 1
- Garlic, finely minced: 2 cloves
- Ground cumin: 1 teaspoon
- Turmeric, ground: 1/2 teaspoon
- Paprika: 1/2 teaspoon
- Season according to your liking with salt and black pepper
- Olive oil: 2 tablespoons
- Cilantro or perhaps parsley, fresh (an optional touch for garnish)

How to Prepare:

✓ Chickpea Choreography: Begin by laying the chickpeas on a bowl. With the artistry of a fork or potato masher, softly crush the chickpeas while preserving some in their original form for a dance of textures.

✓ Onion Overture: In the amphitheater of a skillet, summon the warmth of olive elixir under a medium flame. Include the onions and garlic in this performance, allowing them to sway for 2-3 minutes until the onions adopt a crystalline veil.

✓ Pepper Performance & Spice Serenade: Welcome the bell pepper slices to join the dance and let them cook for a bit. As their dance progresses, shower them with the aromatic notes of cumin, turmeric, paprika, salt, and black pepper. Stir with passion, ensuring the spices dress every element.

✓ Chickpea Chorus: Allow the chickpeas to join the skillet. Mix and let them dance together for 5-7 minutes, harmonizing the flavors.

✓ Verdant Finale: As the performance nears its end, adorn the dish with a sprinkle of verdant cilantro or parsley, offering both a visual and flavorful encore.

✓ Culinary Curtain Call: Present the Chickpea Scramble standalone or as the star of a sandwich or wrap. Relish in the harmonious blend of textures and melodies of taste!

Nutritional Info: Calories: 284 kcal, Protein: 9g, Carbohydrates: 36g, Dietary Fiber: 9g, Sugars: 6g, Fat: 12g, Saturated Fat: 1g, Cholesterol: 0mg, Sodium: 547mg, Potassium: 498mg

---

8. Cranberry Walnut Scones

(Ready in: 15 minutes | Cook Duration: 15-18 min | Persons: 8 scones)

Necessary Items:

- All-purpose flour: 2 cups
- Sugar, granulated: 1/4 cup

- Baking powder: 2 1/2 teaspoons
- Salt: 1/2 teaspoon
- Butter, unsalted, cold and in cube form: 1/2 cup
- Cranberries, dried: 1/2 cup
- Walnuts, chopped: 1/2 cup

- Milk, either whole or 2%: 1/2 cup
- Egg, large: 1
- Vanilla extract: 1 teaspoon
- Orange, just the zest (a delightful optional touch): 1
- Sugar, for a gentle sprinkle on top (only if you wish)

How to Prepare:

✓ Oven Prelude: Ignite the warmth of your oven, dialing its temperament to a steadfast 400°F (200°C). Adorn a baking tray with parchment paper, setting the stage for our gastronomic performance.

✓ Mélange Mastery: In the esteemed basin of a mixing bowl, merge the time-honored ingredients: all-purpose flour, granulated sugar, baking powder, and a touch of salt. With the finesse of a whisk, unify these elements, evoking their combined prowess.

✓ Butter Rhapsody: Usher in the cold, cubed butter to harmonize this culinary symphony. With a pastry cutter's artistry or your fingers' delicate ballet, incorporate the butter, aiming for a texture reminiscent of fine breadcrumbs.

✓ Cranberry & Walnut Waltz: Introduce the sun-dried cranberries and the finely-hewn walnuts, ensuring they are intricately intertwined within the powdery tapestry.

✓ Liquid Sonata: In a separate vessel, orchestrate a blend of milk's richness, an egg, vanilla's whisper, and if you're so inclined, the aromatic zest of an orange.

✓ Harmonious Union: Marry the liquid notes with the powdery composition, pouring the concoction into the floury embrace. Stir with intention but with a gentle hand, ensuring the dough binds.

✓ Sculpting Serenade: On a plan lightly dusted with flour, unveil your dough. With minimal kneading, mold it into a circular tableau, about 1 inch in stature.

✓ Triangular Treasures: Using a sharp-edged instrument (or a bench scraper), segment this masterpiece into 8 equally delectable sections, each promising a bite of ecstasy.

✓ Golden Odyssey: Place these sections on the parchment theater, slightly spaced. If you desire, garnish them with a shimmer of sugar. Commit them to the oven's embrace for 15-18 minutes until they achieve a gilded radiance and clean tales (via toothpick tests).

✓ Epilogue of Elegance: Once their dance in the heat concludes, allow these illustrious scones a respite on the cooling pedestals for a moment's breath. Then, indulge in the artistry of your Cranberry Walnut Scones.

Nutritional Info: Calories: 329 kcal, Protein: 5g, Carbohydrates: 38g, Dietary Fiber: 2g, Sugars: 13g, Fat: 18g, Saturated Fat: 8g, Cholesterol: 55mg, Sodium: 381mg, Potassium: 186mg

9. Pumpkin Spice Oatmeal

(Ready in: 5 minutes | Cook Duration: 10 minutes | Persons: 2)

Necessary Items:

- Rolled oats, old-fashioned style: 1 cup
- Milk, either dairy or a non-dairy variant such as almond or oat: 2 cups

- Pumpkin puree from a can: 1/2 cup
- Maple syrup (adjust according to your sweet tooth): 2 tablespoons

- Pumpkin pie spice (or consider a blend of cinnamon, nutmeg, and cloves): 1 teaspoon

- Salt: 1/4 teaspoon

- Pecans or perhaps walnuts, chopped (an optional touch for the top): 1/4 cup

- Maple syrup or honey, for an extra drizzle (only if you fancy)

- Berries, fresh, or banana slices (a delightful optional garnish)

How to Prepare:

✓ Oats and Milk Matinée: In the embrace of a polished saucepan, combine the old-fashioned rolled oats and milk, initiating their gentle union.

✓ Pumpkin Prelude: To this duet, introduce the rich undertones of canned pumpkin puree, the soft lilt of maple syrup, the aromatic chords of pumpkin pie spices, and a hint of sea salt. Ensure these ingredients meld into a cohesive gastronomic symphony.

✓ Simmering Serenade: Position the saucepan under medium heat, anticipating the first notes of a gentle boil. Once the rhythm sets in, dial down the heat, allowing the composition to simmer for 7-10 minutes. Stir occasionally, observing the oats thicken into a creamy consistency.

✓ Harmonic Honeyed Notes: For those with a penchant for sweeter harmonies, consider an encore of maple syrup or a drizzle of honey.

✓ Garnishing Overture: In your chosen breakfast bowls, ladle the spiced oatmeal. Garnish with the nutty overtones of pecans or walnuts. For a fresh interlude, feature a medley of vibrant berries or the mellow notes of sliced bananas.

✓ Culinary Crescendo: Behold, your Pumpkin Spice Oatmeal opus! Revel in the warmth and texture of this autumn-inspired dish, savoring every spoonful of morning magic.

Nutritional Info: Calories: 285 kcal, Protein: 11g, Carbohydrates: 48g, Dietary Fiber: 6g, Sugars: 15g, Fat: 6g, Saturated Fat: 1g, Cholesterol: 12mg, Sodium: 342mg, Potassium: 325mg

10. Fruit and Nut Muffins

(Ready in: 15 minutes | Cook Duration: 20 min | Persons: 12 muffins)

Necessary Items:

- All-purpose flour: 1 1/2 cups

- Whole wheat flour: 1/2 cup

- Sugar, granulated: 1/2 cup

- Baking powder: 2 teaspoons

- Baking soda: 1/2 teaspoon

- Salt: 1/2 teaspoon

- Butter, unsalted, melted and then cooled: 1/2 cup

- Eggs, large: 2

- Greek yogurt, plain: 1 cup

- Vanilla extract: 1 teaspoon

- Mixed dried fruits (like raisins, cranberries, or apricots): 1/2 cup

- Nuts, chopped (be it walnuts, almonds, or your preference): 1/2 cup

- Orange, just the zest (an optional touch for added zestiness): 1

How to Prepare:

- ✓ Oven's Gentle Call: Initiate the warm embrace of your oven, setting its heart to a cozy 375°F (190°C). Adorn your muffin tin with elegant paper casings or lightly gloss them with butter, ensuring our culinary gems glide out effortlessly.
- ✓ Dry Ingredient Ensemble: In the grand amphitheater of your sturdiest bowl, bring together the classic all-purpose flour, rustic whole wheat counterpart, crystalline sugar, the rising agents of baking powder & soda, and a dash of salt. Allow them to coalesce in an elegant mix.
- ✓ Elixir of Creaminess: In a nearby vessel, blend the velvety melted butter, vivacious eggs, luscious Greek yogurt, and a hint of vanilla's aromatic whisper. Marvel as they unite in a silken concoction.
- ✓ Majestic Merger: Delicately pour the creamy blend into the assembly of dry ingredients, intertwining their characters until they mirror a unified texture. Caution: Overmixing may disturb their composition.
- ✓ Nature's Bounty: Infuse the batter with cherished additions like sun-dried fruits, nature's nutty crunch, and, if the mood beckons, the zesty embrace of an orange.
- ✓ Noble Portioning: Gracefully dispense the crafted mixture into the awaiting muffin casings, filling them to a generous two-thirds, ensuring uniformity in every dwelling.
- ✓ Golden Transformation: Commend the muffin mold to the oven's gentle caress for approximately 18-20 minutes. Patiently anticipate their metamorphosis, confirming their readiness with a wooden probe's clean exit.
- ✓ Momentary Respite: After their golden color arrives, grant the muffins a brief moment of tranquility within their mold, soon guiding them to the airy haven of a cooling rack.
- ✓ Dawn's Delicacy: Presenting your artisanal Fruit and Nut Muffins! Perfect as a morning's embrace or an afternoon's delight, these muffins promise an epicurean experience in every bite.

Nutritional Info: Calories: 230 kcal, Protein: 5g, Carbohydrates: 29g, Dietary Fiber: 2g, Sugars: 13g, Fat: 11g, Saturated Fat: 5g, Cholesterol: 51mg, Sodium: 237mg, Potassium: 120mg

11. Peaches and Cream

(Ready in: 10 minutes | Persons: 2)

Necessary Items:

- Peaches, ripe and sliced: 2
- Greek yogurt: 1/2 cup
- Honey or perhaps maple syrup: 2 tablespoons
- Granola (only if you fancy a crunch): 1/4 cup
- Mint leaves, fresh (a delightful optional garnish)

How to Prepare:

- ✓ Peach Perfection: Initiate your culinary journey by tenderly cleansing the peaches. Honor their natural beauty by delicately peeling or choosing to retain their rustic allure. Carve them into refined segments.
- ✓ Sweet Elixir Blend: In the gentle embrace of a bowl, fuse the velvety Greek yogurt with nature's sweet elixir, be it honey or maple syrup. Stir seamlessly, ensuring they unite in a smooth serenade.
- ✓ Tiered Presentation: Select your glasses or classic bowls. Embark on this gastronomic art by laying a base of the sweetened yogurt.

- ✓ Golden Interlude: Arrange the sculpted peach pieces atop the yogurt, allowing them to nestle seamlessly.
- ✓ Lyrical Layering: Continue this rhythmic dance of yogurt and peaches, crafting layers that resonate with elegance, until you reach the vessel's zenith or the ingredients offer their curtain call.
- ✓ Granola Encore: Should the ensemble beckon a textured finale, let the granola cascade in a crunchy overture atop the yogurt.
- ✓ Minted Accolade: Garnish with vibrant mint leaves, adding a touch of verdant freshness and panache.
- ✓ Chilled Reverie: Entrust your Peach Parfait to the cool of the refrigerator for approximately 30 minutes, allowing flavors to meld in harmonious union.
- ✓ Culinary Reveal: Present your artful Peach and Cream in its cooled magnificence. Savor the layered delight as a sunrise greeting or a midday gourmet respite.

Nutritional Info: Calories: 163 kcal, Protein: 7g, Carbohydrates: 32g, Dietary Fiber: 3g,, Sugars: 28g, Fat: 1g, Saturated Fat: 0g, Cholesterol: 2mg, Sodium: 27mg, Potassium: 308mg

12. Cinnamon Raisin Toast

(Ready in: 5 minutes | Cook Duration: 5 minutes | Persons: 2)

Necessary Items:

- Bread, whole-grain (or your preferred type), sliced: 4 slices

- Butter, unsalted, or perhaps coconut oil: 2 tablespoons

- Cinnamon, ground: 2 teaspoons

- Raisins: 2 tablespoons

- Honey (only if you wish a drizzle): 2 tablespoons

- Berries or fresh fruit (a delightful optional garnish)

How to Prepare:

✓ Preheat Toaster: Plug in your toaster and set it to the desired toasting level.

✓ Butter the Bread: Spread a thin layer of unsalted butter or coconut oil evenly on each slice of bread.

✓ Sprinkle Cinnamon: Sprinkle ground cinnamon over the buttered slices. Adjust the amount to your taste preferences.

✓ Add Raisins: Sprinkle raisins evenly over the slices. Press them gently into the bread to help them stick.

✓ Toast: Place the prepared bread slices into the toaster. Toast until the bread is crispy and slightly golden. The exact toasting time may vary depending on your toaster settings.

✓ Optional Drizzle: If desired, drizzle honey lightly over the toasted slices for added sweetness.

✓ Garnish: Garnish with fresh berries or fruit for a burst of flavor and color.

✓ Serve: Enjoy your Cinnamon Raisin Toast while it's warm and crisp.

Nutritional Info: Calories: 175 kcal, Protein: 3g, Carbohydrates: 26g, Dietary Fiber: 3g, Sugars: 9g, Fat: 7g, Saturated Fat: 4g, Cholesterol: 15mg, Sodium: 144mg, Potassium: 159mg

13. Egg and Cheese Quesadilla

(Ready in: 10 minutes | Cook Duration: 10 minutes | Persons: 2)

Necessary Items:

- Eggs, large: 4
- Milk: 1/4 cup
- Season as per your preference with salt and pepper
- Tortillas, whole-wheat and small: 4
- Cheddar cheese, shredded: 1 cup
- Bell peppers, diced (be it red, green, or a mix): 1/2 cup
- Onions, finely diced: 1/2 cup
- Tomatoes, diced: 1/2 cup
- Olive oil: 2 tablespoons
- Cilantro leaves, fresh (a delightful optional garnish)

How to Prepare:

- ✓ Egg Preparation: In a preferred mixing bowl, whisk together eggs, milk, salt, and pepper. Ensure each ingredient is seamlessly integrated for a unified blend.
- ✓ Tortilla Base: Spread out your tortillas, each primed to embrace an array of flavors. Garnish two tortillas generously with shredded cheddar, setting the stage for their delicious counterparts.
- ✓ Sautéed Veggies: In a skillet over medium heat, warm a drizzle of olive oil. Once heated, introduce bell peppers and onions, sautéing until they soften, typically 3-4 minutes. Towards the end, fold in the diced tomatoes, allowing them to meld for an additional 1-2 minutes.
- ✓ Scrambled Fusion: Combine your previously blended eggs with the sautéed vegetables in the skillet. Gently scramble until the eggs are soft and fully integrated with the veggies.
- ✓ Quesadilla Assembly: Onto your cheese-laden tortillas, spread the scrambled egg mixture evenly. Top with the remaining tortillas, forming a delightful layered medley.
- ✓ Golden Finish: Clean your skillet briefly, then return it to medium heat. Carefully place each quesadilla into the skillet, cooking each side for 2-3 minutes or until they attain a golden hue and the cheese is melt-in-your-mouth luscious.
- ✓ Serving Touch: After a brief pause, deftly slice the quesadillas into halves or neat quarters. A scattering of freshly chopped cilantro provides a vibrant garnish.
- ✓ Dining Delight: Admire your handiwork for a moment, and then indulge in the rich flavors of your Eggs and Cheese Quesadilla Delight. Bon appétit!

Nutritional Info: Calories: 380 kcal, Protein: 18g, Carb: 22g, Dietary Fiber: 3g, Sugars: 5g, Fat: 25g, Saturated Fat: 10g, Cholesterol: 299mg, Sodium: 488mg, Potassium: 297mg

14. Apricot Almond Bites

(Ready in: 15 minutes | Persons: 12 bites)

Necessary Items:

- Apricots, dried: 1 cup
- Almonds: 1 cup
- Coconut, unsweetened and shredded: 1/4 cup

- Honey (only if you fancy a touch of sweetness): 1 tablespoon
- Vanilla extract (an optional flavor enhancer): 1/2 teaspoon
- A subtle hint of salt

How to Prepare:

- ✓ Ingredient Preparation: Begin by organizing all your ingredients. Ensure your apricots are pit-free for a smooth culinary journey.
- ✓ Blending Beginnings: In your food processor, combine the dried apricots, almonds, shredded coconut, honey (if available), vanilla extract (if using), and a pinch of salt.
- ✓ Processing Perfection: Pulse the ingredients until they come together to form a cohesive, slightly sticky mixture. The ideal consistency should hold together when pressed between your fingers.
- ✓ Forming Fancies: With clean hands, scoop out small portions of the mixture. Shape them into your preferred forms, whether that be bite-sized balls or compact squares.
- ✓ Chilling Chamber: Place your apricot-almond creations in the refrigerator to set for around 30 minutes. This step ensures they firm up nicely.
- ✓ Serving and Storing: Once set, present them as delightful treats for immediate consumption. Any leftovers can be stored in an airtight container in the refrigerator, ready to be enjoyed throughout the week. Dive in and savor the delightful combination of flavors!

Nutritional Info: Calories: 79 kcal, Protein: 2g, Carbohydrates: 10g, Dietary Fiber: 2g, Sugars: 7g, Fat: 4g, Saturated Fat: 0g, Cholesterol: 0mg, Sodium: 1mg, Potassium: 175mg

15. Nut Butter and Banana Sandwich

(Ready in: 5 minutes | Persons: 1)

Necessary Items:

- Bread, whole-grain, sliced: 2 slices

- Nut butter, pick your favorite (like almond, peanut, or cashew): 2 tablespoons

- Banana, ripe and sliced: 1

- Honey (only if you fancy a drizzle): 1/2 teaspoon

- Cinnamon (a delightful optional sprinkle): a hint

How to Prepare:

- ✓ Ingredient Line-up: Begin by setting all your ingredients on the countertop.
- ✓ Nut Butter Layering: On one slice of your whole-grain bread, spread a generous layer of your preferred nut butter, ensuring even coverage.
- ✓ Banana Placement: Neatly arrange the banana slices atop the nut butter to create a delicious layer.
- ✓ Sweetness Swirl (Optional): If you're in the mood for some extra sweetness, give the bananas a delicate drizzle of honey.
- ✓ Cinnamon Spritz (Optional): Enhance the taste profile by lightly dusting the banana layer with cinnamon.
- ✓ Final Assembly: Crown your creation with the second slice of whole-grain bread, pressing down gently.

✓ Presentation Cut: For easier enjoyment, cut the sandwich into two halves with a sharp knife, and voilà! Your delightful sandwich is ready to be savored.

Nutritional Info: Calories: 350 kcal, Protein: 7g, Carbohydrates: 50g, Dietary Fiber: 8g, Sugars: 19g, Fat: 16g, Saturated Fat: 2g, Cholesterol: 0mg, Sodium: 300mg, Potassium: 470mg

16. Egg Muffins

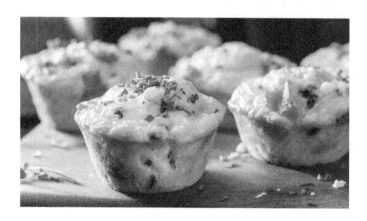

(Ready in: 10 minutes | Cook Duration: 20 minutes | Persons: 6)

Necessary Items:

- Eggs, large: 6
- Milk or perhaps a non-dairy variant: 1/4 cup
- Bell peppers, any hue, diced: 1/2 cup
- Tomatoes, finely diced: 1/2 cup
- Onions, chopped: 1/4 cup
- Spinach or maybe kale, diced (an optional green touch): 1/4 cup
- Cheese, shredded (pick your preference, such as cheddar or mozzarella): 1/2 cup
- Season according to your liking with salt and pepper
- Cooking spray or muffin liners for ease of preparation.

How to Prepare:

✓ Oven Prelude: Prepare your oven to a welcoming 350°F (175°C), laying down the red carpet for our egg muffin debut.

✓ Setting the Stage: Deck out your 6-slot muffin tray with a spritz of non-stick spray or by fitting each slot with chic muffin liners, ensuring a smooth entrance and exit for our sweet.

✓ Egg Symphony: In a revered mixing vessel, break open the eggs to release their potential. With deliberate strokes, marry them with the milk, seasoning with a whisper of salt and a flirt of pepper.

✓ Veggie Cast Call: Populate each muffin mold with our veggie ensemble: vibrant bell peppers, luscious tomatoes, pungent onions, and verdant spinach. Allow them their diva moments by ensuring a balanced cast in each mold.

✓ Egg Lagoon Creation: Gently cascade the whisked egg mixture over the waiting veggies, filling each nook and cranny up to 3/4 full.

✓ Cheese Finale: As the crescendo nears, shower each mold with a generous flurry of shredded cheese, promising a golden encore.

- ✓ Oven Performance: Usher the muffin tray into the oven's spotlight, letting our stars dazzle and rise for about 20 minutes until they sport a sun-kissed glow.
- ✓ Applause Moment: Upon their triumphant exit, allow them a moment's rest. When ready, introduce them to your eagerly awaiting plate and relish the gourmet spectacle with each bite!

Nutritional Info: Calories: 130 kcal, Protein: 9g, Carbohydrates: 4g, Dietary Fiber: 1g, Sugars: 2g Fat: 9g, Saturated Fat: 3g, Cholesterol: 195mg, Sodium: 150mg, Potassium: 170mg

17. Cottage Cheese with Pineapple

(Ready in: 5 minutes | Persons: 2)

Necessary Items:

- Cottage cheese, low-fat: 1 cup
- Pineapple, fresh and diced: 1/2 cup
- Honey (only if you fancy a touch of sweetness): 1 tablespoon
- Cinnamon (a delightful optional sprinkle): a hint

How to Prepare:

- ✓ Pineapple Selection: Handpick your protagonist – a ripe and radiant pineapple. Carve and craft it into delightful bite-sized morsels.
- ✓ Culinary Theater: Seize your mixing bowl – this is where the culinary ballet unveils. Allow the velvety, low-fat cottage cheese to waltz with the pineapple chunks.
- ✓ Golden Nectar Touch (Optional): For an added touch of sweetness, bestow a golden drizzle of honey upon the pairing. Adjust to your palate's preference.
- ✓ Cinnamon Whispers (Optional): Elevate the ensemble with a hint of warm cinnamon, enhancing the depth of their dance.
- ✓ The Blend Ballet: Gently stir and unite the components in a synchronized ballet until their dance feels seamless.
- ✓ Curtain Call: Divide this gourmet performance between two serving dishes and savor the medley at its freshest peak!

Nutritional Info: Calories: 150 kcal, Protein: 14g, Carb: 16g, Dietary, Fiber: 1g, Sugars: 14g, Fat: 3g, Saturated Fat: 1.5g, Cholesterol: 15mg, Sodium: 400mg, Potassium: 190mg

18. Cherry Almond Smoothie

(Ready in: 5 minutes | Persons: 2)

Necessary Items:

- Almond milk, unsweetened: 1 cup
- Cherries, frozen: 1 cup
- Greek yogurt, low-fat: 1/2 cup
- Almond butter: 1 tablespoon
- Honey (only if you wish a touch of sweetness): 1 tablespoon
- Ice cubes (an optional chill factor): a handful
- Almonds, sliced (a delightful optional garnish)

How to Prepare:

- ✓ Culinary Prelude: Assemble your gourmet ensemble, ensuring each ingredient is poised for a culinary concerto.
- ✓ Blend Ballet: Into the blending chamber, introduce the silky almond milk, followed by the rich chorus of frozen cherries. Next, invite the velvety Greek yogurt, a hint of almond butter, and, for a touch of sweetness, a drizzle of golden honey.
- ✓ Frosty Intermezzo (Optional): For a colder crescendo, scatter in a few ice crystals to heighten the refreshment.
- ✓ Crescendo Mix: Secure the blending chamber's lid and initiate the whirlwind waltz, ensuring each component merges in harmonious unity.
- ✓ Duet Decant: Pour the Cherry Almond aria into twin crystal chalices, revealing its rich hue and consistency.
- ✓ Garnish Grace Note (Optional): Adorn the top with delicate almond slivers, adding a crisp contrast to your beverage ballet.

Nutritional Info: Calories: 180 kcal, Protein: 9g, Carbohydrates: 25g, Dietary, Fiber: 3g, Sugars: 19g, Fat: 6g, Saturated Fat: 0.5g, Cholesterol: 2mg, Sodium: 115mg, Potassium: 230mg

19. Quinoa Breakfast Bowl

(Ready in: 10 minutes | Cook Duration: 15 minutes | Persons: 2)

Necessary Items:

- Quinoa: 1 cup
- Water: 2 cups
- Almond milk or another milk of your preference: 1 cup
- Honey or perhaps maple syrup: 2 tablespoons
- Vanilla extract: 1 teaspoon
- Fresh berries, mixed (like strawberries, blueberries, or raspberries): 1 cup
- Nuts, chopped (consider almonds or walnuts): 1/4 cup
- Chia seeds: 2 tablespoons
- Cinnamon (a delightful optional sprinkle): a hint

How to Prepare:

- ✓ Quinoa Purification: Begin by lavishing your quinoa with a crisp rinse, ensuring any residual bitterness is thoroughly dispatched.
- ✓ Culinary Steambath for Quinoa: Immerse the purified quinoa into a pot with two cups of water, inviting it to bask in a bubbling simmer. Once the miniature cauldrons form, reduce the heat and allow the quinoa to gently cook under a veil until it has absorbed the water and achieved a tender, fluffy disposition, approximately 15 minutes. Allow a moment's respite before proceeding.
- ✓ Almond Milk Elixir: In a separate vessel, gently warm the almond milk, and sweeten the mixture with honey or maple syrup, enhanced with a splash of vanilla essence. Stir to intertwine the flavors harmoniously, and then allow it to rest momentarily.
- ✓ Elegant Plating: Distribute the rested quinoa amongst two serving bowls, and gently cascade your sweetened almond milk elixir over each.
- ✓ Garnishing Gems: Embellish your quinoa beds with an array of fresh berries, a scatter of robust nuts, a sprinkle of chia seeds, and, should you desire, a delicate dusting of cinnamon to elevate the ensemble.

✓ Gastronomic Delight: Enjoy your Quinoa Breakfast Bowl in its comforting warmth and commence your day with this nutrient-dense delight. May your morning be as splendid as your breakfast!

Nutritional Info: Calories: 350 kcal, Protein: 9g, Carbohydrates: 56g, Dietary, Fiber: 8g, Sugars: 18g, Fat: 11g, Saturated Fat: 1g, Cholesterol: 0mg, Sodium: 60mg, Potassium: 446mg

---

20. Oatmeal with Nuts

(Ready in: 5 minutes | Cook Duration: 10 minutes | Persons: 2)

Necessary Items:

- Oats, old-fashioned: 1 cup

- Water: 2 cups

- Milk, pick your favorite (like almond, soy, or dairy): 1 cup

- Nuts, mixed and chopped (consider almonds, walnuts, or pecans): 1/4 cup

- Honey or perhaps maple syrup (adjust according to your sweet tooth): 2 tablespoons

- Cinnamon, ground (an optional touch for flavor): 1/2 teaspoon

- Fresh fruit slices (like bananas or berries) for a delightful top

- A subtle hint of salt.

How to Prepare:

✓ Oat Ritual: Immerse your old-fashioned oats into a cauldron of simmering water, seasoned with a pinch of salt. Ignite the heat beneath them, allowing the liquid to bubble. As the ebullience calms, let the oats indulge in their rich bath for a tender 5-7 minutes, absorbing and transforming into a creamy concoction.

✓ Creamy Cadence: Introduce your preferred milk to the simmering oats, creating a delicate infusion. Continue the gentle stir, weaving the ingredients together for another 2-3 minutes.

✓ Syrupy Serenades and Cinnamon Chords: Allow honey or maple syrup to trickle in, adding layers of melodious sweetness. For those seeking a spicy undertone, a sprinkle of cinnamon can elevate the orchestra.

✓ Nutty Nocturne: On a neighboring platform (skillet), let the assortment of chopped nuts waltz. With medium heat as their guide, they'll pirouette, releasing an intoxicating aroma within a span of 2-3 minutes. Be vigilant, for their performance can be swift and fleeting!

✓ Opulent Overture: Arrange two bowls as the audience chamber and cascade the luscious oat mixture into them. Crown with the pirouetting nuts and a medley of vibrant fruit embellishments.

✓ Gastronomic Ovation: Delight in the embrace of your Rich and Nutty Oat Ensemble. While applause might be silent, the satiation will resonate loud and clear!

Nutritional Info: Calories: 300 kcal, Protein: 9g, Carbohydrates: 40g, Dietary, Fiber: 5g, Sugars: 10g, Fat: 12g, Saturated Fat: 2g, Cholesterol: 6mg, Sodium: 60mg, Potassium: 240mg

Chapter 5: Lunch Recipes For Intermittent Fasting

1.Teriyaki Salmon with Steamed Broccoli

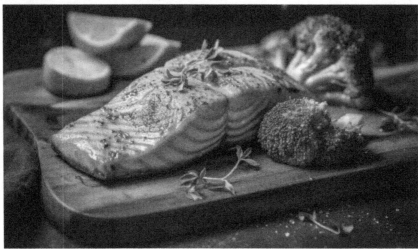

(Ready in: 10 mins | Cook Duration: 15 mins | Persons: 2)

Necessary Items:

- Salmon fillets: 2
- Teriyaki sauce: 1/4 cup
- Honey: 2 tablespoons
- Soy sauce, low-sodium: 1 tablespoon
- Garlic, finely minced: 2 cloves
- Ginger, fresh and minced: 1 teaspoon
- Broccoli florets: 2 cups
- Sesame seeds (a delightful touch for garnish)
- Green onions (for a fresh garnish)

How to Prepare:

- ✓ Sauce Craftsmanship: Skillfully whisk together the teriyaki sauce, sweet honey, rich soy sauce, aromatic minced garlic, and invigorating minced ginger in a modest bowl, conjuring a delightful gastronomic harmony.
- ✓ Salmon Marination: Tenderly cradle your salmon fillets in a shallow dish and serenade them with half of your exquisitely crafted sauce. Allow them to marinate, absorbing the vibrant flavors for about 10 minutes, while reserving the remaining sauce for a later encore.
- ✓ Baking the Salmon: Set your oven to a welcoming 375°F (190°C). Gently place your marinated salmon fillets onto a parchment-lined or lightly greased baking sheet, allowing them to perform solos for 12-15 minutes until they yield gracefully to a fork's inquiry. For a smoky outdoor alternative, consider using the grill.
- ✓ Broccoli's Steamed Waltz: Concurrently, allow your broccoli florets to twirl in a gentle steam for a lively yet brief 5-minute dance, ensuring they retain their vibrant hue and crisp texture, whether under a traditional steamer or within the quick embrace of a microwave.
- ✓ Sauce's Encore: In a discreet saucepan, grant the remaining teriyaki sauce mixture a gentle warming over low heat, preparing it for its second act.

✓ Plating Elegance: Present the brightly steamed broccoli on your choicest plate, gently nestling the oven-kissed salmon atop. Lavish them with the warm teriyaki sauce, allowing it to cascade gracefully over the ensemble.

✓ Garnish with Finesse: As a concluding act, cascade a shower of sesame seeds and a scattering of fresh green onion slices, bestowing zest and visual appeal. The stage is yours—savor the Teriyaki Salmon and Broccoli medley and bask in the ovation of your palate!

Nutritional Info: Calories: 350 kcal Protein: 30g, Carbohydrates: 22g, Dietary Fiber: 3g, Sugars: 15g, Fat: 15g, Saturated Fat: 3g, Cholesterol: 80mg, Sodium: 900mg, Potassium: 750mg

2. Roasted Red Pepper Hummus Wrap

(Ready in: 15 mins | Persons: 2)

Necessary Items:

- Tortillas, whole-grain or spinach, large: 2

- Hummus, roasted red pepper variant: 1 cup

- Spinach leaves, fresh: 1 cup

- Cucumber, finely sliced: 1/2 cup

- Red bell pepper, finely sliced: 1/2 cup

- Carrots, shredded: 1/2 cup

- Red onion, thinly cut: 1/4 cup

- Feta cheese, crumbled (an optional touch of tang): 1/4 cup

- Season according to your liking with salt and pepper.

How to Prepare:

✓ Pristine Palette: Position your tortillas elegantly on your workspace or chosen platter, as untouched canvases eagerly anticipating an artful touch.

✓ Hummus Hues: Brush a generous spread of the roasted red pepper hummus across each tortilla canvas, ensuring you leave a modest, thumb-width frame around the edges, allowing the tortilla's natural hue to peek through.

✓ Vegetable Vivacity: On this luscious foundation, lay down a verdant carpet of fresh spinach leaves. Onto this, add bold strokes of crisp cucumber, vibrant strips of red bell pepper, delicate threads of carrot, and concentric loops of red onion. For an artisanal touch, sprinkle the canvas with the crumbled jewels of feta cheese.

✓ Whispers of Season & Delicate Roll: Infuse the colors with subtle hints of salt and pepper, echoing the complexity of nature. Then, with gentle care, fold the tortilla's sides inward and roll from bottom to top, encapsulating your creation with grace.

✓ Masterful Cuts: With deliberate and artful motion, segment each wraps diagonally, unveiling the radiant interior layers, each telling a unique tale of flavor and texture.

✓ Culinary Exhibition: Serve your Roasted Red Pepper Hummus Wraps immediately in their radiant glory or wrap them in parchment or foil, reminiscent of cherished art pieces, ideal for a gourmet journey or picnic affair.

Nutritional Info: Calories: 330 kcal, Protein: 10g, Carbohydrates: 41g, Dietary Fiber: 8g, Sugars: 6g, Fat: 15g, Saturated Fat: 2g, Cholesterol: 0mg, Sodium: 620mg, Potassium: 500mg

3. Seared Tofu with Peanut Sauce

(Ready in: 15 minutes | Cook Duration: 10 mins| Persons: 2)

Necessary Items:

For the Tofu Delight:

- Extra-firm tofu, pressed and cubed: 1 block (14 oz)
- Soy sauce or perhaps tamari (for those avoiding gluten): 2 tablespoons
- Sesame oil: 1 tablespoon
- Garlic powder: 1/2 teaspoon
- Ginger powder: 1/2 teaspoon
- Vegetable oil (to achieve that perfect sear): 1 tablespoon

For the Nutty Sauce:

- Peanut butter, creamy: 1/4 cup
- Soy sauce or tamari (again, gluten-free friendly): 2 tablespoons
- Maple syrup or honey: 2 tablespoons
- Rice vinegar: 1 tablespoon
- Sesame oil: 1 teaspoon
- Garlic powder: 1/2 teaspoon
- Ginger powder: 1/2 teaspoon
- Warm water (to get the right consistency): 2-3 tablespoons

To Plate:

- Brown rice or quinoa, cooked to perfection
- Broccoli florets, steamed
- Green onions, finely chopped (a fresh garnish)
- Peanuts, crushed (an optional crunch)
- Lime wedges (for that zesty finish)

How to Prepare:

For Seared Tofu:

- ✓ Tofu's Tantalizing Tango: Elegantly introduce your tofu to a sensuous blend of soy sauce, hints of sesame, and aromatic nuances of garlic and ginger. Allow them to be engrossed in this affair for a dedicated 10 minutes, soaking up every aromatic note.
- ✓ Tofu's Graceful Debut: In a skillet set under medium-high fuel, drizzle a hint of vegetable oil. Present your marinated tofu, allowing it to pirouette to a rich golden embrace, approximately 2-3 minutes per facet. Once their cooking is complete, escort them to a cooling rest.

For Peanut Sauce:

- ✓ Concocting a Culinary Concerto: With precision, meld peanut butter, soy's deep undertones, sweet symphonies of maple syrup or honey, piquant notes of rice vinegar, sesame's rich undertones, and the harmonious duet of garlic and ginger powders. For a velvety texture, usher in warm water, a tablespoon at each interlude, tuning the sauce to perfection.

Assembling the Culinary Performance:

✓ The Grand Presentation: Cast a comforting quantity of warm brown rice or quinoa onto two exquisite plates, forming the primary stage.

✓ Tofu's Grand Re-entry: On this prepared platform, let your golden tofu and vibrant steamed broccoli make their dramatic entrance, standing side by side in their gastronomic glory.

✓ Peanut Sauce Serenade: Lavishly drape your ingredients with meticulously crafted peanut sauce, ensuring every element is accentuated with its luxurious touch.

✓ Culinary Coda: For an impeccable finish, scatter emerald fragments of chopped greens and specks of crushed peanuts. Bestow lime crescents on the side, offering a zesty encore for the eager palate.

Nutritional Info: Calories: 380 kcal, Protein: 19g, Carbohydrates: 17g, Dietary Fiber: 3g, Sugars: 10g, Fat: 29g, Saturated Fat: 5g, Cholesterol: 0mg, Sodium: 822mg, Potassium: 337mg

4. Chicken and Vegetable Kebabs

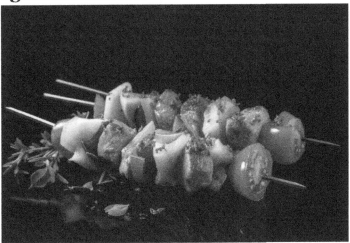

(Ready in: 20 mins | Cook Duration: 15 mins | Persons: 4)

Necessary Items:

• Chicken breasts, boneless and skinless, cubed into 1-inch pieces: 1 pound

• Red bell pepper, chunked: 1

• Green bell pepper, chunked: 1

• Red onion, chunked: 1

• Zucchini, sliced into rounds: 1

• Cherry tomatoes: 8-10

• Olive oil: 1/4 cup

• Garlic, minced: 2 cloves

• Dried oregano: 1 teaspoon

• Dried thyme: 1 teaspoon

• Salt and pepper: to your liking

• Wooden skewers (remember to soak them in water for about 30 minutes to prevent burning)

How to Prepare:

- ✓ Dressing Decantation: In the spirit of culinary tradition, combine the olive oil, aromatic hints of garlic, fragrant oregano, and thyme, seasoned with salt and pepper in a mixing vessel (or bowl). This dressing will imbue both chicken and vegetables with an irresistible allure.
- ✓ Chicken Marinade Meditation: Bathe the chicken cubes in this fragrant concoction, either in a practical marinating pouch (resealable plastic bag) or a marinating dish. Introduce them to half of the dressing, allowing them to marinate in this bath. Let them rest and infuse in the refrigerator for about 15 minutes, or longer if deeper flavors are desired.
- ✓ Vegetable Veneration: Assemble your chosen assembly of vegetables—bell peppers, red onion, zucchini, and cherry tomatoes—and dress them gracefully with the remaining marinade in another bowl, ensuring each piece is elegantly coated.
- ✓ Skewer Craftsmanship: Heat your grill to a robust medium-high temperature. With a craftsman's precision, thread the marinated chicken and dressed vegetables onto your pre-soaked skewers (wooden or metal), harmonizing the colors and tastes.
- ✓ Grill's Embrace: Present your artful kebabs to the warm embrace of the grill. Allow them to sear for 5-7 minutes on each side until the chicken is thoroughly cooked and the vegetables have a tender-crisp finish, bearing the hallmark of char. Rotate intermittently to achieve an even golden hue.
- ✓ Gastronomic Gala: After their dance on the grill, let your kebabs rest momentarily. Then, serve them forth, and let all partake in the savory spectacle you've crafted!

Nutritional Info: Calories: 285 kcal, Protein: 26g, Carbohydrates: 11g, Dietary Fiber: 2g, Sugars: 5g, Fat: 15g, Saturated Fat: 2g, Cholesterol: 68mg, Sodium: 73mg, Potassium: 619mg

5. Ratatouille with Quinoa

(Ready in: 15 mins | Cook Duration: 30 mins | Persons: 4)

Necessary Items:

- Quinoa: 1 cup
- Water: 2 cups
- Olive oil: 2 tablespoons
- Chopped onion: 1
- Minced garlic: 3 cloves
- Red bell pepper, diced: 1
- Yellow bell pepper, diced: 1
- Diced eggplant: 1
- Zucchinis, diced: 2
- Diced tomatoes (including juice) from a 14 oz can
- Dried thyme: 1 teaspoon
- Dried oregano: 1 teaspoon
- Salt and pepper: to your preference
- Optional: Fresh basil leaves for garnishing.

How to Prepare:

- ✓ Quinoa's Preparation: Begin by rinsing the quinoa under a cool cascade to freshen its essence. In its dedicated pot, submerge it in 2 cups of fresh water. Turn up the flame until the water approaches a boil, then moderate it to a soft simmer, sealing the vessel with a lid. Allow the quinoa to absorb and swell for 15 minutes. Once this communion is complete, unveil and fluff the grains with finesse using a fork. Reserve for the final act.

- ✓ Foundation of Flavors: In the expansive domain of a skillet, introduce the lustrous olive oil, warming it under medium heat. Introduce the aromatic duo of onion and garlic. Saute them until they convey their translucent glow, typically in 2-3 minutes.
- ✓ Vegetable Medley: Usher in the vibrant brigade - bell peppers in sunset hues, robust eggplant, and lively zucchini. Engage them in a saute, stirring and mingling for about 5-7 minutes until they start to soften.
- ✓ Herbaceous Infusion: Incorporate the diced tomatoes, brimming with their natural nectar. Season with the timeless herbs - thyme and oregano, then balance with salt and pepper. Diminish the heat, secure the skillet with its lid, and allow the medley to meld and intensify over 15-20 minutes. Periodically, taste and adjust seasonings to perfect their symphony.
- ✓ Culinary Showcase: Onto your chosen serving dishes, spread the prepared quinoa. Over this, ladle generous servings of the Ratatouille. For a touch of freshness, garnish with sprigs or torn leaves of basil.

Nutritional Info: Calories: 318 kcal, Protein: 7g, Carbohydrates: 56g, Dietary Fiber: 9g,, Sugars: 9g, Fat: 9g, Saturated Fat: 1g, Cholesterol: 0mg, Sodium: 487mg, Potassium: 1230mg

6. Lemon Garlic Shrimp Skewers

(Ready in: 15 mins | Cook Duration: 6-8 mins | Persons: 4)

Necessary Items:

- Large shrimp (peeled and deveined): 1 pound
- Olive oil: 2 tablespoons
- Minced garlic: 3 cloves
- Lemon zest from 1 lemon
- Fresh lemon juice from 1 lemon
- Dried oregano: 1 teaspoon
- Salt and pepper: to your preference
- Pre-soaked wooden skewers (soak for 30 minutes).

How to Prepare:

- ✓ Citrus-Marinated Shrimp: Start by combining olive oil, finely minced garlic, freshly grated lemon zest, and its tangy juice, along with aromatic dried oregano in a bowl. Season this marinade with salt and pepper and mix until harmonious. Immerse the shrimp in this lively concoction, ensuring each piece is well-coated. Let the shrimp marinate, absorbing the flavors for approximately 10 minutes.
- ✓ Prepping the Shrimp: Gently thread each shrimp onto pre-soaked wooden skewers, giving each its rightful space to ensure even cooking.
- ✓ Grill Preparation: Preheat your grill to a robust medium-high. Make sure the grill grates are clean, then lightly oil them to prevent the shrimp from sticking during cooking.
- ✓ Grilling the Shrimp: Carefully place the marinated shrimp skewers on the grill. Cook for about 2-3 minutes on each side or until the shrimp achieve a radiant pink hue, signifying they're cooked to perfection. Be attentive, as shrimp can cook quickly and it's essential not to overcook them.
- ✓ Serving the Dish: Transfer the perfectly grilled shrimp skewers to a serving platter. For a final touch, garnish with some additional lemon zest or a sprinkle of freshly chopped herbs.

Nutritional Info: Calories: 182 kcal, Protein: 23g, Carbohydrates: 2g, Dietary Fiber: 0g, Sugars: 0g, Fat: 9g, Saturated Fat: 1g, Cholesterol: 191mg, Sodium: 180m, Potassium: 144mg

7. Asparagus and Mushroom Risotto

(Ready in: 10 mins | Cook Duration: 30 mins | Persons: 4)

Necessary Items:

- Arborio rice: 1 cup
- Low-sodium vegetable broth: 4 cups
- Asparagus segments (2-inch length): 1 cup
- Sliced mushrooms (cremini or shiitake recommended): 1 cup
- Finely diced onion: 1 small
- Minced garlic: 2 cloves
- Optional: dry white wine: 1/2 cup
- Olive oil: 2 tablespoons
- Grated Parmesan cheese: 1/2 cup
- Season with salt and pepper as desired
- Optional garnish: fresh parsley leaves.

How to Prepare:

✓ Beginning with the Broth: Warm your vegetable broth gently in a saucepan over low heat. Keep this comforting foundation simmering, ensuring it's ready to embrace the other ingredients as the process unfolds.

✓ Sauteing the Vegetables: In a spacious skillet, heat the olive oil over a medium setting. Add the onions, allowing them to soften and turn translucent, a process taking about 2-3 minutes. Introduce garlic for its aromatic contribution, followed by the mushrooms, cooking until they're richly golden.

✓ Adding the Rice: Fold in the Arborio rice, ensuring it's well-coated with the oil and vegetable mixture. Stir continuously, letting the rice grains turn translucent around the edges.

✓ White Wine Reduction (Optional): If using white wine, pour it in, stirring consistently. Allow most of the liquid to evaporate, leaving behind its flavorful essence.

✓ Building the Risotto: Start incorporating the simmering broth, one ladle at a time, into the rice mixture. Continuously stir, ensuring each broth addition is nearly absorbed before adding the next. This careful process will take around 18-20 minutes, resulting in a rich and creamy risotto texture.

✓ Incorporating the Asparagus: About 10 minutes into the risotto's cooking time, add the asparagus pieces, letting them cook and meld with the risotto, achieving a tender texture.

✓ Finishing Touches: Once the risotto is velvety and the asparagus tender, remove from heat. Fold in the Parmesan cheese, enriching the risotto, and season to taste.

✓ Serving the Dish: Dish out your creamy risotto immediately while hot. Garnish with freshly chopped parsley, adding a vibrant touch to your culinary creation.

Nutritional Info: Calories: 330 kcal, Protein: 9g, Carbohydrates: 51g, Dietary Fiber: 3g, Sugars: 3g, Fat: 8g, Saturated Fat: 2g, Cholesterol: 9mg, Sodium: 770mg, Potassium: 323mg

8. Greek Lemon Chicken Soup (Avgolemono)

(Ready in: 15 mins | Cook Duration: 30 mins | Persons: 4)

Necessary Items:

- Low-sodium chicken broth: 4 cups
- Boneless, skinless chicken breasts: 2
- Orzo pasta: 1/2 cup
- Large eggs: 3

- Freshly squeezed lemon juice: from 2 lemons
- Freshly chopped dill: 1/4 cup

- Season according to preference: salt and pepper
- Lemon slices and sprigs of dill

How to Prepare:

- ✓ Chicken Poaching: Start your Greek culinary expedition by gently heating a pot of chicken broth over medium heat. Gently lower the chicken breasts into this simmering liquid, letting them poach until fully cooked, roughly 15-20 minutes. Once done, use a couple of forks to shred the chicken into bite-sized pieces.
- ✓ Orzo Cooking: With the chicken set aside, introduce the orzo pasta into the same broth, allowing it to cook until al dente, approximately 8-10 minutes.
- ✓ Preparing the Egg-Lemon Mix: In a separate bowl, whisk together the eggs and lemon juice until well combined, creating a smooth and velvety mixture.
- ✓ Tempering the Eggs: To prevent the eggs from curdling when introduced to the hot broth, gently mix in a ladle of the hot broth into the egg-lemon mixture, whisking constantly. This step acclimatizes the mixture to the warmth.
- ✓ Integrating the Mixtures: Gradually pour the tempered egg-lemon blend into the pot with the orzo, stirring constantly. The soup will become rich and slightly creamy in texture.
- ✓ Incorporating the Chicken: Add the shredded chicken back into the pot, along with chopped dill. Season to taste with salt and pepper, ensuring a well-balanced flavor.
- ✓ Simmering: Let the entire concoction simmer for an additional 5 minutes, making sure all ingredients meld and infuse together.
- ✓ Serving: Serve the Avgolemono (Greek Lemon Chicken Soup) hot in bowls, garnished with a slice of lemon and a sprig of fresh dill. Enjoy this Grecian delight and savor the rich combination of flavors.

Nutritional Info: Calories: 245 kcal, Protein: 25g, Carbohydrates: 17g, Dietary Fiber: 1g, Sugars: 1g, Fat: 8g, Saturated Fat: 2g, Cholesterol: 162mg, Sodium: 120mg, Potassium: 330mg

9. Sweet Potato and Black Bean Tacos

(Ready in: 15 min | Cook Duration: 25 min | Persons: 4)

Necessary Items:

For the Filling:

- Diced sweet potatoes (medium-sized): 2
- Black beans (15 oz can), drained and rinsed: 1 can
- Finely diced red onion: 1 small
- Minced garlic: 2 cloves

- Chili powder: 1 teaspoon
- Ground cumin: 1/2 teaspoon
- Smoked paprika: 1/2 teaspoon
- Olive oil: 2 tablespoons
- Season with salt and pepper as desired

For Assembly:

- Corn or whole wheat tortillas (small-sized): 8

Optional Toppings:

- Salsa, avocado slices, shredded lettuce, chopped cilantro, and lime wedges for garnish.

How to Prepare:

- ✓ Roasted Sweet Potato Prep: Prepare the oven to a sturdy 425°F (220°C). As the oven gains heat, prep your baking sheet for action. Toss the sweet potato cubes in olive oil, and season generously with chili powder, cumin, smoked paprika, salt, and pepper. Ensure they are evenly coated, then spread them out on the baking sheet. Roast these cubes for about 20-25 minutes or until they are perfectly crispy yet tender.
- ✓ Sautéed Bean Foundation: Concurrently, on a stovetop, heat a skillet and drizzle in a tablespoon of olive oil. To this, add the finely chopped garlic and red onion, sautéing them until the onion becomes translucent, which should take around 3-4 minutes.
- ✓ Black Bean Mix: Introduce the black beans to the skillet, seasoning them with salt and pepper to taste. Cook everything together for about 5 minutes, melding the flavors. If you prefer a partially mashed texture, press down on some of the beans with the back of a fork.
- ✓ Tortilla Warm-up: Ready your tortillas by gently heating them in the skillet or microwave, each for about 20 seconds or until they're soft and pliable.
- ✓ Taco Compilation: Once all elements are prepped, it's time to assemble your tacos. Begin by laying down a base of the roasted sweet potatoes on each tortilla. Follow up with the black bean mixture. Top these layers with your choice of salsa, slices of ripe avocado, shredded lettuce, a sprinkle of cilantro, and a zest of lime.
- ✓ Serving Time: Once assembled, serve these Sweet Potato and Black Bean Tacos immediately. Enjoy the delicious medley of flavors with every bite!

Nutritional Info: Calories: 350 kcal, Protein: 8g, Carbohydrates: 59g, Dietary Fiber: 10g, Sugars: 8g, Fat: 10g, Saturated Fat: 2g, Cholesterol: 0mg, Sodium: 445mg, Potassium: 738mg

10. Turkey and Avocado Lettuce Wraps

(Ready in: 15 minutes | Cook Duration: 10 minutes | Persons: 4)

Necessary Items:

- Turkey, ground: 1 pound
- Finely chopped onion: 1 small
- Minced garlic: 2 cloves
- Cumin, ground: 1 teaspoon
- Chili powder: 1 teaspoon
- Paprika: 1/2 teaspoon
- Salt and pepper: to your preference
- Avocado, sliced: 1 large
- Lettuce leaves (like iceberg or Romaine): 8 large
- Optional toppings: salsa, shredded cheese, diced tomatoes, fresh cilantro, and lime wedges for serving.

How to Prepare:

- ✓ Turkey Sauté: In a skillet over medium-high heat, crumble and cook the ground turkey until it turns a deep golden brown. Stir consistently to ensure even cooking.
- ✓ Addition of Aromatics: To the browned turkey, incorporate the finely chopped onion and minced garlic. Continue to sauté the mixture until the onion becomes translucent and the turkey is fully cooked, ensuring flavors meld.
- ✓ Seasoning Mix: Enhance the skillet's contents by seasoning with ground cumin, chili powder, paprika, salt, and pepper. Stir well, ensuring the spices coat the turkey uniformly. Allow this mixture to cook for another 2-3 minutes for flavors to marry, then remove from heat.

- ✓ Lettuce Preparation: Lay out the crisp lettuce leaves on your countertop, ready to be filled with the seasoned turkey mixture.
- ✓ Avocado Layer: Place slices of creamy avocado over the turkey, lending a rich contrast to the savory filling.
- ✓ Toppings Galore: For added layers of flavor and texture, feel free to garnish your wraps with extras like salsa, shredded cheese, freshly chopped tomatoes, a sprinkle of cilantro, or even a squeeze of lime juice.
- ✓ Assemble the Wraps: Carefully fold the lettuce leaves around the filling, ensuring they are secure and ready to be savored.
- ✓ Serve Promptly: Bring these delectable lettuce wraps to the table while fresh and enjoy the satisfied reactions from your guests.

Nutritional Info: Calories: 250 kcal, Protein: 27g, Carbohydrates: 7g, Dietary Fiber: 3g, Sugars: 2g, Fat: 13g, Saturated Fat: 2g, Cholesterol: 62mg, Sodium: 87mg, Potassium: 677mg

11. Thai-Inspired Vegetable Curry

(Ready in: 15 minutes | Cook Duration: 25 minutes | Persons: 4)

Necessary Items:

- Vegetable oil: 1 tablespoon
- Onion, finely chopped: 1 small
- Garlic, minced: 2 cloves
- Thai red curry paste: 1 tablespoon
- Coconut milk (14 ounces can)
- Vegetable broth: 1 cup
- Mixed vegetables (like bell peppers, broccoli, carrots, snap peas): 2 cups
- Optional protein: diced tofu or cooked chickpeas (1 cup)
- Soy sauce or tamari: 1 tablespoon
- Brown sugar or coconut sugar: 1 tablespoon
- Lime juice: from 1 lime
- Optional garnish: fresh cilantro leaves
- Serving suggestion: cooked rice or cauliflower rice.

How to Prepare:

- ✓ Preparation of Vegetables: Begin by meticulously cleaning your selection of fresh vegetables. Once cleaned, chop them uniformly, ensuring they are bite-sized and ready for cooking.
- ✓ Sauté Base: In a spacious skillet, warm the vegetable oil over medium heat. As it shimmers, add the diced onions, allowing them to soften and turn translucent. Once achieved, add the minced garlic, cooking briefly until aromatic but not browned.
- ✓ Adding Thai Flavors: Mix in the Thai red curry paste, ensuring it integrates seamlessly with the onions and garlic, infusing the oil with its rich, spicy profile.
- ✓ Liquid Ingredients: Slowly incorporate the creamy coconut milk along with the hearty vegetable broth into the skillet. Stir continuously, ensuring the curry paste melds into the liquids, resulting in a smooth base for your curry.
- ✓ Vegetables and Protein: Introduce the chopped vegetables to the simmering curry base. If using tofu or chickpeas, add them now. Let the mixture simmer until the vegetables are tender and the curry has thickened to your preferred consistency, roughly 10-15 minutes.

✓ Seasoning and Balancing Flavors: To balance the curry's flavors, stir in the soy sauce or tamari for depth, brown sugar for a hint of sweetness, and a squeeze of fresh lime juice for acidity. Taste and adjust the seasoning to your preference.

✓ Serving: Spoon the rich Thai vegetable curry over a bed of freshly steamed rice or a lighter alternative like cauliflower rice. Garnish with freshly chopped cilantro for a burst of freshness before serving.

Nutritional Info: Calories: 250 kcal, Protein: 6g, Carbohydrates: 16g, Dietary Fiber: 4g, Sugars: 6g, Fat: 20g, Saturated Fat: 14g, Cholesterol: omg, Sodium: 500mg, Potassium: 460mg

---

12. Zucchini Noodles with Pesto

(Ready in: 15 minutes | Cook Duration: 5 minutes | Persons: 2)

Necessary Items:

- Zucchinis, medium-sized: 2
- Fresh basil leaves: 1 cup
- Pine nuts: 1/4 cup
- Parmesan cheese, grated: 1/4 cup
- Garlic cloves: 2
- Extra-virgin olive oil: 1/4 cup
- Salt and pepper: according to your preference
- Optional garnish: cherry tomatoes
- Optional topping: additional grated Parmesan cheese

How to Prepare:

✓ Preparation of Zucchini Noodles: Using a spiralizer or julienne peeler, carve the zucchini into noodle-like strands. Lay them out on a paper towel to absorb excess moisture and set aside.

✓ Pesto Preparation: In a food processor, combine fresh basil leaves, pine nuts, Parmesan cheese, and garlic cloves. Blend until the mixture is finely processed.

✓ Adding Oil to Pesto: With the food processor running, drizzle in the extra-virgin olive oil in a steady stream. This will create a smooth, unified sauce. Taste and season with salt and pepper, adding more oil if necessary for desired consistency.

✓ Cooking the Zucchini: Heat a splash of olive oil in a large skillet over medium heat. Once hot, add the zucchini noodles, tossing and cooking them for 2-3 minutes, just until they're slightly softened but still maintain a slight crunch.

✓ Combining Zucchini and Pesto: Pour the freshly made pesto over the zucchini noodles, mixing well to coat each strand. Allow them to cook together for an additional 1-2 minutes.

✓ Serving: Transfer the zucchini noodles coated in pesto to serving dishes. Garnish with halved cherry tomatoes and a generous sprinkle of grated Parmesan cheese before serving.

Nutritional Info: Calories: 320 kcal, Protein: 7g, Carbohydrates: 10g, Dietary Fiber: 3g, Sugars: 3g, Fat: 30g, Saturated Fat: 5g, Cholesterol: 8mg, Sodium: 240mg, Potassium: 580mg

13. Roasted Butternut Squash and Chickpea Bowl

(Ready in: 15 minutes | Cook Duration: 30 minutes| Persons: 2)

Necessary Items:

- Butternut squash, cubed: 2 cups
- Chickpeas (15 oz can), drained and rinsed: 1 can
- Olive oil: 2 tablespoons
- Ground cumin: 1 teaspoon
- Smoked paprika: 1/2 teaspoon
- Salt and pepper: according to your preference

- Quinoa, cooked: 2 cups
- Baby spinach leaves: 2 cups
- Optional topping: crumbled feta cheese, 1/4 cup
- Optional garnish: pomegranate seeds, 1/4 cup
- Optional drizzle: tahini dressing

How to Prepare:

✓ Oven Warm-up: Let your oven to a temperature of 400°F (200°C), preparing it for the roasting session ahead.

✓ Squash & Chickpea Preparation: In a large mixing bowl, combine butternut squash cubes, chickpeas, olive oil, cumin, and smoked paprika. Toss until the squash and chickpeas are well-coated in the seasonings.

✓ Roasting: Spread the seasoned squash and chickpeas onto a baking sheet lined with parchment paper, ensuring they're spaced apart for even cooking. Roast in the preheated oven for about 25-30 minutes, or until the squash becomes tender and the chickpeas turn slightly crispy.

✓ Serve with Quinoa: Begin by placing a layer of cooked quinoa in your serving bowls, creating a base.

✓ Assemble: Over the quinoa, arrange the roasted butternut squash and chickpeas. Add a handful of fresh baby spinach leaves.

✓ Garnishing Touch: Sprinkle the bowls with crumbled feta cheese and pomegranate seeds, adding texture and color to the dish.

✓ Finishing Drizzle: Drizzle a generous amount of tahini dressing over the bowls to add a creamy richness to the dish.

✓ Serve and Enjoy: Bring your prepared bowls to the table and enjoy a nutritious and delightful meal!

Nutritional Info: Calories: 450 kcal, Protein: 11g, Carbohydrates: 70g, Dietary Fiber: 12g, Sugars: 5g, Fat: 16g, Saturated Fat: 2g, Cholesterol: 0mg, Sodium: 350mg, Potassium: 842mg

14. Caprese Chicken Salad

(Ready in: 15 minutes | Cook Duration: 15 minutes - for chicken, if not using precooked chicken - | Persons: 2)

Necessary Items:

- Chicken breasts, boneless and skinless: 2 pieces (alternatively, rotisserie chicken can be used)

- Olive oil: 1 tablespoon
- Salt and pepper: according to your preference

- Cherry tomatoes, cut in half: 2 cups

- Bocconcini (small mozzarella balls): 1 cup

- Fresh basil, torn or finely chopped: 1/4 cup

- Baby spinach or arugula: 2 cups

- For drizzling: Balsamic glaze

- For added flavor: Extra virgin olive oil drizzle

- Optional enhancement: Balsamic reduction drizzle

How to Prepare:

✓ Chicken Preparation: If using rotisserie chicken, have it ready. Alternatively, season chicken breasts with salt and black pepper. In a skillet over medium-high heat, add olive oil and cook the chicken breasts for approximately 6-7 minutes on each side, or until they reach an internal temperature of 165°F (74°C). Once cooked, set aside and allow them to rest before slicing them.

✓ Salad Base: In a large salad bowl or on individual serving plates, lay a generous bed of baby spinach or arugula, depending on your preference.

✓ Caprese Assembly: Distribute cherry tomatoes, slices of fresh mozzarella, and basil leaves evenly over the greens, creating a visually appealing and flavorful combination.

✓ Add the Chicken: Place the rotisserie or freshly cooked and sliced chicken on top of the salad, making it the star of the dish.

✓ Dressing Application: Drizzle a blend of extra virgin olive oil and balsamic glaze over the salad. Alternatively, you can use a balsamic reduction for a richer flavor profile.

✓ Seasoning Adjustments: Taste and adjust the seasoning if needed, adding additional salt or pepper to enhance the flavors.

✓ Serve: Present your Caprese Chicken Salad immediately and enjoy the harmonious blend of ingredients!

Nutritional Info: Calories: 400 kcal, Protein: 36g, Carbohydrates: 9g, Dietary Fiber: 2g, Sugars: 5g, Fat: 25g, Saturated Fat: 11g, Cholesterol: 115mg, Sodium: 450mg, Potassium: 550mg

15. Stuffed Bell Peppers with Quinoa and Feta

(Ready in: 20 minutes | Cook Duration: 45 minutes | Persons: 4)

Necessary Items:

- Bell peppers of any hue: 4 large pieces

- Quinoa, thoroughly rinsed: 1 cup

- Vegetable broth or alternatively, water: 2 cups

- Feta cheese, crumbled: 1 cup

- Cherry tomatoes, finely diced: 1/2 cup

- Fresh spinach, finely chopped: 1/2 cup

- Red onion, finely chopped: 1/4 cup

- Garlic, minced: 2 cloves

- Olive oil: 2 tablespoons

- Dried oregano: 1 teaspoon

- Salt and black pepper: as per your preference

- Fresh basil leaves: a few pieces

How to Prepare:

✓ Stage Setup: Light up your oven stage to a warm 375°F (190°C), letting it get ready for the upcoming performance.

- ✓ Bell Pepper Preparations: Imagine the bell peppers as delicate vases and gently snip off their crowns. Delicately, yet confidently, scoop out their inner secrets (seeds and membranes).
- ✓ Quinoa Dance: Waltz into the world of quinoa. In your trusted saucepan, let the vegetable broth (or water) reach its boiling crescendo. Introduce the rinsed quinoa, then allow the heat to mellow, covering it to simmer. After about a 15-minute dance, let it rest, fluffing it up for its next act.
- ✓ Filling Harmony: Picture a grand mixing bowl as the gathering arena. Parade in the poised quinoa, lively feta, vibrant cherry tomatoes, verdant spinach, zesty red onion, aromatic garlic, timeless oregano, and smooth olive oil. Season with dashes of salt and pepper, and then let them all mingle and harmonize.
- ✓ Bell Pepper Ensembles: Like dressing a star for the main act, gracefully fill the bell peppers with the quinoa ensemble, ensuring each layer nestles comfortably.
- ✓ Oven Ballet: Place your prepared performers (bell peppers) in their baking theatre. Veil them with aluminum foil, a gentle shield, and let them pirouette in the oven for 30-35 minutes until they attain tender perfection.
- ✓ Curtain Call: As the bell pepper stars exit the oven stage, bestow upon them a sprinkle of fresh basil leaves.

Nutritional Info: Calories: 390 kcal, Protein: 12g, Carbohydrates: 47g, Dietary Fiber: 6g, Sugars: 7, Fat: 18g, Saturated Fat: 6g, Cholesterol: 25mg, Sodium: 640mg, Potassium: 742mg

16. Mediterranean Tuna and White Bean Salad

(Ready in: 15 minutes | Persons: 4)

Necessary Items:

- Tuna, drained from water (5 oz cans): 12 cans
- Cannellini beans, rinsed and drained (15 oz cans): 2 cans
- Cherry tomatoes, sliced in half: 1 cup
- Cucumber, diced: 1/2 cup
- Red onion, finely diced: 1/4 cup
- Kalamata olives, pitted and chopped: 1/4 cup
- Fresh parsley, finely chopped: 1/4 cup
- Dried oregano: 1 teaspoon
- Extra-virgin olive oil: 2 tablespoons
- Red wine vinegar: 2 tablespoons
- Salt and black pepper: as per your preference

For Garnishing (Optional):

- Feta cheese, crumbled: a handful

How to Prepare:

- ✓ Setting the Stage: Envision your large mixing bowl as the grand arena. Parade in the mighty tuna, having been drained and given a flaky texture, the trusty cannellini beans, vivacious cherry tomatoes sliced in their prime, crisp cucumber cubes, red onion finely sculpted, Kalamata olives in their sleek sliced attire, and the evergreen fresh parsley.
- ✓ Dressing Serenade: In an intimate smaller bowl, let the melodious extra-virgin olive oil waltz with the vibrant red wine vinegar. Introduce them to the aromatic dried oregano,

with dashes of salt and black pepper to set the rhythm. Whisk them into a harmonious blend.

- ✓ Ensemble Crescendo: Shower the salad performers with the dressing serenade. Embrace the flavors, letting them mingle and dance, ensuring everyone gets a touch of the harmonious dressing.
- ✓ Interlude: Cloak your salad masterpiece and grant it a cooling retreat in the refrigerator. A 30-minute pause lets the flavors converse and bond. As the finale, let feta cheese crumbles take the spotlight for that encore presentation.

Nutritional Info: Calories: 350 kcal, Protein: 28g, Carbohydrates: 36g, Dietary Fiber: 9g, Sugars: 3g, Fat: 11g, Saturated Fat: 2g, Cholesterol: 35mg, Sodium: 680mg, Potassium: 685mg

17. Cauliflower and Broccoli Casserole with Cheese

(Ready in: 20 minutes | Cook Duration: 30 minutes | Persons: 4-6)

Necessary Items:

- Cauliflower, separated into florets: 1 head
- Broccoli, separated into florets: 1 head
- Olive oil: 2 tablespoons
- Onion, finely diced: 1 small
- Garlic, minced: 2 cloves
- Cheddar cheese, shredded: 1 cup
- Parmesan cheese, grated: 1/2 cup
- Sour cream: 1/2 cup
- Mayonnaise: 1/2 cup
- Dijon mustard: 1 teaspoon
- Dried thyme: 1/2 teaspoon
- Salt and black pepper: as per your preference
- Breadcrumbs: 1/2 cup
- Fresh parsley, finely chopped: a handful

How to Prepare:

- ✓ Oven's Awakening: Awaken your oven to a cozy 350°F (175°C). Ready a 9x13-inch baking vessel with a light brush of grease.
- ✓ Vegetable Spa: Immerse the broccoli and cauliflower warriors into a boiling bath, letting them relax and rejuvenate for 3-4 minutes. Once they've achieved that perfectly al dente texture, drain them and let them bask in their glory.
- ✓ Cheese Magic Potion: In your cauldron (or large skillet), summon the olive oil's powers over a medium flame. Introduce finely crafted onion and garlic to the mix, letting them dance and mingle until the onion dons a sheer translucent veil. Turn the flame to a gentle whisper and beckon the cheddar and Parmesan spirits, followed by the sour cream, mayonnaise, mystical Dijon, thyme whispers, and the ever-trusted salt and pepper guardians. Stir until a smooth, enchanting potion is formed.
- ✓ Vegetable and Cheese Union: In the prepared baking vessel, let the refreshed vegetables lay in harmony. Serenade them with the cheese potion, making sure every nook and cranny is bathed in its richness.
- ✓ Crisp Finale: Should you desire, let a rain of breadcrumbs grace the top, promising a delightful crunch.
- ✓ Oven's Embrace: Entrust the casserole to the oven's warmth for about 25-30 minutes. The casserole shall emerge bubbling with joy; its top kissed golden by the oven.
- ✓ Final Flourish: After a brief moment of rest, adorn this majestic creation with fresh parsley confetti and serve as the crowning glory of your feast.

Nutritional Info: Calories: 450 kcal, Protein: 16g, Carbohydrates: 18g, Dietary Fiber: 5g, Sugars: 6g, Fat: 36g, Saturated Fat: 12g, Cholesterol: 50mg, Sodium: 550mg, Potassium: 690mg

18. Caramelized Onion and Goat Cheese Frittata

(Ready in: 15 minutes | Cook Duration: 25 minutes | Persons: 4-6)

Necessary Items:

- Olive oil: 1 tablespoon
- Onions, large and thinly sliced: 2
- Eggs, large: 8
- Milk: 1/4 cup

- Seasoning: Salt and black pepper, as per your liking
- Goat cheese, crumbled: 4 ounces
- Garnish: Fresh parsley, chopped, 2 tablespoons

How to Prepare:

- ✓ Stage Setup: Warm up the stage (your oven) to a toasty 350°F (175°C).
- ✓ Onion Waltz: In your grand oven-ready skillet, serenade the olive oil over a gentle medium-low tune. Introduce the onion ribbons, letting them sway and twirl until they wear a rich golden gown, about 15-20 minutes of their graceful dance. Let half of these star performers take a bow and exit the stage to a plate on the side.
- ✓ Egg Orchestra: In the green room (mixing bowl), conduct a symphony with eggs and milk, whisking them into a harmonious blend. Sprinkle in some salt and pepper notes to elevate the melody.
- ✓ Grand Ensemble: With the remaining onion dancers still on stage (skillet), pour the orchestrated egg blend over them. A gentle stir ensures every performer knows their place.
- ✓ Goat Cheese Solo: Now, let the goat cheese crumbles take the spotlight, scattering gracefully over the eggy ensemble.
- ✓ Curtain Rise: With everything in place, move your skillet stage to the pre-warmed oven. Let the performance unfold for about 15-20 minutes until our frittata masterpiece stands tall and proud with golden edges.
- ✓ Encore: After a brief cool-down, bring back our onion stars for a final act, along with a sprinkle of fresh parsley confetti. Now, serve this morning showstopper and take a bow!

Nutritional Info: Calories: 280 kcal, Protein: 14g, Carbohydrates: 9g, Dietary Fiber: 2g, Sugars: 4g, Fat: 20g, Saturated Fat: 9g, Cholesterol: 333mg, Sodium: 290mg, Potassium: 251mg

19. Zesty Cucumber and Avocado Gazpacho

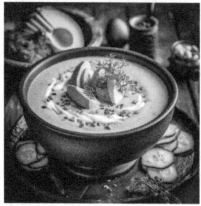

(Ready in: 15 minutes | Persons: 4)

Necessary Items:

- Cucumbers, large, peeled, seeded, and chopped: 2
- Avocados, ripe, peeled, and pitted: 2
- Greek yogurt: 1 cup
- Cilantro, fresh and chopped: 1/4 cup
- Garlic, minced: 2 cloves
- Red onion, finely chopped: 1/4 cup
- Jalapeño pepper, seeded and minced (adjust for spice): 1
- Lime juice, fresh: 2 tablespoons
- Lemon juice, fresh: 2 tablespoons
- Extra-virgin olive oil: 1/4 cup
- Seasoning: Salt and black pepper, to your preference
- Optional for garnish: Additional chopped cilantro, diced avocado, and a splash of olive oil

How to Prepare:

✓ Avocado & Cucumber Prep Station: Embark on your culinary journey by giving the cucumbers a good peel and dice, making sure to discard any seeds. Next, face the mighty avocados, giving them a peel and bidding the pits farewell.

✓ Smoothie-Style Soup Creation: Into the magical vortex of your blender or food processor, summon the prepped cucumber and avocado, followed by Greek yogurt, the aromatic cilantro, a hint of garlic, snippets of red onion, a touch of spirited jalapeño, and the zesty duo of lime and lemon juices. Hit the power and watch them whirl into a creamy dreamscape.

✓ Oil Elixir Drop: With the machine's rhythm ongoing, artistically pour in the golden stream of extra-virgin olive oil, ensuring it becomes one with the verdant blend.

✓ Flavor Meditation: Bless your concoction with the timeless salt and pepper duo. Let it retreat into the cool haven of your fridge, meditating for at least 2 hours, marrying all the flavors in serenity.

✓ The Grand Reveal: As serving time beckons, present this chilled elixir in bowls. Evoke the beauty with adornments of fresh cilantro snippets, avocado cubes, and perhaps an artistic olive oil drizzle. Cheers to a refreshing masterpiece!

Nutritional Info: Calories: 295 kcal, Protein: 5g, Carbohydrates: 16g, Dietary Fiber: 7g, Sugars: 5g, Fat: 25g, Saturated Fat: 4g, Cholesterol: 2mg, Sodium: 61mg, Potassium: 833mg

20. Mango and Shrimp Salad with Chili-Lime Dressing

(Ready in: 20 minutes | Cook Duration: 5 minutes | Persons: 4)

Necessary Items:

For the Main Dish:

- Shrimp, large, peeled and deveined: 1 pound
- Mangoes, ripe, peeled, pitted, and diced: 2
- Cucumber, peeled, seeded, and diced: 1
- Red bell pepper, finely chopped: 1
- Red onion, thinly sliced: 1/2
- Cilantro, fresh and chopped: 1/4 cup
- Mixed greens or spinach: 4 cups

For the Zesty Lime Dressing:

- Lime juice, freshly squeezed: 3 tablespoons
- Extra-virgin olive oil: 2 tablespoons
- Sweetener (honey or maple syrup): 1 tablespoon
- Chili powder (adjust for desired heat): 1 teaspoon
- Seasoning: Salt and black pepper, to your preference

How to Prepare:

For the Salad:

- ✓ Shrimp Tango: Ignite a passionate dance in a generous skillet over a medium-high flame. Let a hint of olive oil sizzle, then invite the shrimp to dance, swirling for about 2-3 minutes on each side. Once they blush a beautiful pink, let them rest and cool off stage.
- ✓ Tropical Medley: While the shrimp takes its pause in a salad coliseum, summon a vibrant ensemble: sun-kissed mango cubes, crisp cucumber bits, radiant red bell pepper chunks, wisps of red onion, and a sprinkle of zesty cilantro.
- ✓ The Grand Assembly: Bring back the star performers – our rested shrimp – and let them dive into the tropical medley. When it's showtime, lay a green carpet of mixed salad leaves or spinach on your desired stage – be it plates or a grand platter – and let the vibrant assembly take the spotlight.

For the Chili-Lime Dressing:

- ✓ Prepare the Dressing: In a small bowl, whisk together the fresh lime juice, extra-virgin olive oil, honey or maple syrup, and chili powder until well combined. Season with salt and black pepper to taste. Adjust the chili powder to your preferred level of spiciness.
- ✓ Dress the Salad: Drizzle the chili-lime dressing over the salad ingredients.
- ✓ Toss and Serve: Gently toss the salad to combine all the ingredients and evenly coat them with the dressing.

Nutritional Info: Calories: 315 kcal, Protein: 20g, Carbohydrates: 33g, Dietary Fiber: 4g, Sugars: 24g, Fat: 12g, Saturated Fat: 1g, Cholesterol: 143mg, Sodium: 195mg, Potassium: 602mg

Chapter 6: Dinner Recipes For Intermittent Fasting

1. Creamy Tomato Basil Soup

(Ready in: 10mins | Cook Duration: 30mins | Persons: 4)

Necessary Items:

- Crushed tomatoes: 1 can (28 ounces)
- Olive oil: 1 tablespoon
- Onion, finely chopped: 1 small
- Garlic, minced: 2 cloves
- Basil, dried: 1 teaspoon
- Oregano, dried: 1 teaspoon
- Red pepper flakes (adjust for heat): 1/2 teaspoon
- Vegetable broth, low-sodium: 1/2 cup
- Almond milk, unsweetened (or milk of choice): 1/2 cup
- Seasoning: Salt and black pepper, to your liking
- Fresh basil leaves for an optional garnish

How to Prepare:

- ✓ A Golden Beginning: Spark a large cauldron to medium warmth and let the olive oil do a graceful waltz. Introduce the onion and let them sway for 3-4 minutes until they glow with a see-through shimmer.
- ✓ Herbal Whispers: Time to serenade the pot with murmurs of garlic, wisps of basil, hints of oregano, and a playful kick of red pepper flakes. Let this aromatic ensemble perform for a minute or two, filling the air with their scentful melodies.
- ✓ Tomato Tango: As the pot's symphony heightens, cascade in the crushed tomatoes and vegetable broth. Stir the pot's contents, leading them to a gentle crescendo, then let them serenely hum together for about 20 minutes, with an occasional stir.
- ✓ Smooth Transformation: With the grace of an immersion blender or the might of a traditional one (working patiently in rounds), morph the concoction into a silky potion.
- ✓ Almond Embrace: Pour the blended masterpiece back into its cauldron and gently fold in the almond milk. Warm their reunion but avoid a boiling frenzy.
- ✓ Taste's Finishing Touch: Whisper salt and black pepper into the mix, adjusting for the perfect harmony.
- ✓ Serving Symphony: Present this luscious tomato-basil creation piping hot, crowned with a flourish of fresh basil. Enjoy the encore!

Nutritional Info: Cal: 110, Total Fat: 4g, Carb: 17g, Dietary Fiber: 4g, Sugars: 8g, Protein: 2g

2. Garlic Butter Shrimp Scampi

(Ready in: 10mins | Cook Duration: 10mins | Persons: 2)

Necessary Items:

- Large shrimp, peeled and deveined: 8 oz
- Linguine or pasta of choice: 4 oz
- Unsalted butter: 2 tablespoons
- Garlic, minced: 3 cloves
- Chicken broth: 1/4 cup
- Juice of 1 lemon

- Fresh parsley, chopped: 2 tablespoons
- Salt and black pepper, to taste
- Grated Parmesan cheese (optional, for garnish)

How to Prepare:

- ✓ Pasta Prelude: Dive into the linguine's world by swirling it in boiling water, letting it sway until it's gracefully al dente. Rescue it from the water, let it catch its breath, and await its grand return.
- ✓ Butter Ballet: In the heart of a vast skillet, let butter pirouette to a melt over medium warmth. Usher in the garlic, allowing it a brief solo of about a minute, filling the stage with its aromatic essence.
- ✓ Shrimp Soiree: Welcome the shrimp to this culinary ballet, letting them take center stage for a mere 1-2 minutes on each side until they don a radiant pink attire. Bid them a brief farewell as they exit the stage.
- ✓ Broth Ballad: On the same seasoned stage, serenade the skillet with chicken broth and zesty lemon drops. Let this duet simmer and reduce to a richer, more intense melody for 2-3 minutes.
- ✓ Grand Reunion: The curtain rises as the shrimp re-enter, accompanied by the linguine. Watch as they all waltz, twirling in the garlic butter embrace, absorbing every note of flavor.
- ✓ Flavor's Finale: Whisper secrets of salt and pepper into the mix. Introduce fresh parsley, causing a final burst of vibrant energy.
- ✓ Encore Presentation: Plate this delightful performance piping hot with a sprinkle of Parmesan snow if your heart so desires.

Nutrition: Cal: 350, Total Fat: 12g, Carb: 30g, Dietary Fiber: 2g, Sugars: 1g, Protein: 30g

3. Spinach and Mushroom Stuffed Pork Tenderloin

(Ready in: 20 minutes | Cook Duration: 30mins | Serving 2)

Necessary Items:

- Pork tenderloin (about 1 pound): 1
- Fresh spinach, chopped: 1 cup
- Mushrooms, finely chopped: 1/2 cup
- Garlic, minced: 2 cloves
- Shredded mozzarella cheese: 1/4 cup
- Olive oil: 2 tablespoons
- Salt and black pepper, to taste
- Cooking twine

How to Prepare:

- ✓ Oven Overtures: Kickstart the culinary concert by firing up your oven to a cozy 375°F (190°C).
- ✓ Garlic Prelude: Glide into a skillet and let a spoon of olive oil waltz in the warmth. Soon after, escort the garlic in and let it serenade the space for a minute, releasing its aromatic aria.
- ✓ Mushroom & Spinach Duet: Welcome the mushrooms, allowing their velvety voices to merge with the garlic's melody for about 3-4 minutes. Just when they've hit the right note, let spinach dance in, shimmering and wilting gracefully. Whisper salt and pepper notes to perfect the harmony.
- ✓ Pork's Solo: Lay the pork tenderloin on center stage, slicing it carefully for a grand butterfly reveal. Sandwich it between protective sheets and tenderly flatten its surface, prepping it for the act ahead.

- ✓ Filling Fantasia: Season the pork's stage with salt and pepper. Layer it with the previously prepared vegetable duet, followed by a mozzarella cascade. Then, with artistic flair, roll the tenderloin, capturing the essence within. Bind this masterpiece with twine, securing every inch of flavor.
- ✓ Golden Encore: Summon another spoon of olive oil in a skillet, ensuring it's oven-ready. Present the pork, letting all sides bask in the golden spotlight for about 3 minutes each.
- ✓ Oven's Grand Performance: The skillet, with its star, takes its position in the oven. Let the pork serenade for about 20-25 minutes or until its core sings at 145°F (63°C). Adjust the act based on your encore preference.
- ✓ Curtain Call: Upon the performance's end, wrap the tenderloin in a foil embrace, allowing it to reflect on its journey for 5-10 minutes.
- ✓ Grand Finale: Release the twine, unveil the tenderloin's tales in luscious slices, and serve to an awaiting audience.

Nutritional Info: Cal: 350, Total Fat: 18g, Carb: 5g, Dietary Fiber: 2g, Sugars: 1g, Protein: 40g

4. Balsamic Glazed Brussels Sprouts

(Ready in: 10 mins | Cook Duration: 20 mins | Persons: 2)

Necessary Items:

- Brussels sprouts, trimmed and halved: 2 cups
- Olive oil: 2 tablespoons
- Balsamic vinegar: 2 tablespoons
- Garlic, minced: 2 cloves
- Salt and black pepper, to taste
- Honey or maple syrup (optional, for sweetness): 1 tablespoon
- Grated Parmesan cheese (optional, for garnish)
- Chopped fresh parsley (optional, for garnish)

How to Prepare:

- ✓ Warming Up: Light up your oven's enthusiasm to a hearty 400°F (200°C).
- ✓ Sprout's Marinade Soiree: Assemble those Brussels sprouts in a mixing arena. Shower them with olive oil, whisper secrets of minced garlic, and splash them with balsamic tales. Let them waltz in salt and pepper rain, ensuring they're dressed uniformly for the ball. For those craving a sweet twist, invite honey or maple syrup to the dance.
- ✓ Sprouts' Stage: Elevate your baking sheet's elegance with a parchment paper carpet. Parade the dressed sprouts across, ensuring they each claim their spotlight.
- ✓ Oven Ovation: Allow the sprouts to revel in the oven's warmth for a 15-20 minute soiree until they sway tenderly with caramelized charm. Dance with them once or twice, ensuring each side experiences the glow.
- ✓ Curtain Close: Once their performance reaches its peak, escort the sprouts to a regal serving platter.
- ✓ Final Flourish: For those seeking additional grandeur, sprinkle them with Parmesan confetti and parsley garnish.
- ✓ Dinner's Star: Present these Balsamic Glazed Brussels Sprouts, now ready to steal the spotlight on your dinner stage.

Nutritional Info: Cal: 180, Total Fat: 11g, Carb: 17g, Dietary Fiber: 5g, Sugars: 6g, Protein: 4g

5. Stuffed Acorn Squash with Quinoa and Cranberries

(Ready in: 15mins | Cook Duration: 50mins | Persons: 2)

Necessary Items:

- Acorn squash, halved and seeds removed: 1
- Quinoa, rinsed: 1/2 cup
- Vegetable broth or water: 1 cup
- Dried cranberries: 1/4 cup
- Chopped pecans or walnuts: 1/4 cup
- Chopped fresh parsley: 1/4 cup
- Ground cinnamon: 1/2 teaspoon
- Salt and black pepper, to taste
- Olive oil for drizzling

How to Prepare:

- ✓ Stage Prep: Ignite your oven's passion to a comforting 375°F (190°C).
- ✓ Squash Prelude: Present the acorn squash halves, like awaiting stages, onto a baking platform. Shower them with olive oil's affection and a gentle whisper of salt and pepper. Gift them a 35-40 minute ballet in the oven's embrace until they yield gracefully to a fork's touch.
- ✓ Quinoa Interlude: Dance the quinoa under a cascading cold waterfall, ensuring a refreshing rinse. Lead the cleansed quinoa into a saucepan ballroom with vegetable broth or water. Raise the tempo to a boil, then waltz to a simmer, cloaking them for a 15-20 minute serenade. Unveil and fluff up the quinoa, now ready for the next act.
- ✓ Quinoa Ensemble: In the mixing chamber, unite the harmonious quinoa, cranberries' sweet notes, crunchy nut rhythms, parsley's fresh choreography, cinnamon's warm embrace, and a touch of salt. Let the ingredients perform their intricate ballet.
- ✓ Squash's Encore: As the acorn squash emerges from the oven's spotlight, cradle the quinoa ensemble into each squash stage, ensuring a gentle yet full embrace.
- ✓ Finale: Grant the stuffed acorn stars another 10-minute performance in the oven, allowing a mingling of flavors and a hint of crispiness on the ensemble's surface.
- ✓ Curtain Call: Once their ovation is done, let the stuffed acorn squash retreat for a brief cooling interlude.
- ✓ Standing Ovation: For a final flourish, shower them with parsley's encore. Now, present the Acorn Squash & Quinoa Symphony to your awaiting audience.

Nutritional Info: Calories: 380, Fat: 11g, Carb: 67g, Dietary Fiber: 10g, Sugars: 11g, Protein: 9g

6. Garlic-Herb Roasted Cod with Cherry Tomatoes

(Ready in: 10mins | Cook Duration: 20mins Persons: 2)

Necessary Items:

- Cod fillets (6-8 oz each): 2
- Cherry tomatoes: 1 pint
- Garlic cloves, minced: 4
- Fresh basil, chopped: 2 tablespoons
- Fresh parsley, chopped: 2 tablespoons
- Olive oil: 2 tablespoons
- Salt and black pepper, to taste
- Lemon wedges for garnish

How to Prepare:

- ✓ Oven's Warm Embrace: Set your oven's ambiance to a toasty 400°F (200°C).

- ✓ Tomato Ballet: Dive into the mixing arena with cherry tomatoes, aromatic garlic whispers, basil's fresh waltz, parsley's green jig, and the luxurious glide of olive oil. Let them sway and swirl to a harmony of salt and pepper, ensuring every tomato is embraced.
- ✓ Cod's Stage Setup: Lay your pristine cod performers on a parchment-papered stage (baking sheet), and sprinkle them with the classic duo – salt and pepper – preparing them for the spotlight.
- ✓ Tomato Serenade: With elegance, let the tomato ensemble serenade the cod, blanketing them with their herb-rich melody.
- ✓ Oven Ovation: Let the cod and its accompaniment dance in the oven's warmth for about 15-20 minutes. The curtain falls when the cod elegantly flakes at the touch of a fork, and the tomatoes put on a soft and slightly sunburnt show.
- ✓ Finishing Flourish: As the performance concludes, accentuate the dish with a zesty lemon encore.
- ✓ Pairing Suggestions: This Garlic-Herb Roasted Cod's performance pairs beautifully with the gentle rustle of steamed greens or the crisp applause of a light salad.

Nutritional Info: Calories: 290, Fat: 12g, Carb: 8g, Dietary Fiber: 2g, Sugars: 4g, Protein: 36g

7. Grilled Lemon Herb Tofu Steaks

(Ready in: 30 minutes - including marinating time - | Cook Duration: 10 mins | Persons: 2)

Necessary Items:

- Extra-firm tofu (14 oz block): 1
- Olive oil: 2 tablespoons
- Lemon (zest and juice): 1
- Garlic cloves, minced: 2
- Fresh parsley, chopped: 2 tablespoons
- Dried oregano: 1 teaspoon
- Salt and black pepper, to taste
- Lemon wedges for garnish

How to Prepare:

- ✓ Tofu's Spa Day: Begin by pampering your tofu. Tuck it between two plush kitchen towels or paper comforters. Add a weighty companion like a cast-iron skillet to gently squeeze out its worries (excess moisture) for a soothing 20-minute session.
- ✓ Herb Symphony: As tofu unwinds, conjure up a zesty potion. Dance a whisk through olive oil, spirited lemon zest, lemon's zesty elixir, whispers of garlic, fresh parsley twirls, oregano's magic, and the timeless duo of salt and pepper in a cozy bowl.
- ✓ Tofu Transformation: Once reenergized, carve the tofu into twin majestic steaks.
- ✓ Marinade Bath: Nestle the tofu twins in a dish, showering them with the prepared zesty potion. Ensure each side is luxuriously coated. Let them soak in the flavors, flipping midway in a 10-15 minute aromatic interlude.
- ✓ Grill's Warm Embrace: Wake up your grill or grill pan to a medium-high passion. For those using a grill pan, dress it lightly in oil to make the dance smooth.
- ✓ Tofu's Fiery Waltz: Glide the tofu on the grill, letting it sway for 4-5 minutes on each side until it wears charred stripes and its inner warmth is rekindled.
- ✓ Restful Respite: Once their dance concludes, let the tofu steaks recline for a brief moment.
- ✓ Dress for the Feast: Adorn with lemon crescents and a sprinkle of verdant parsley.

✓ Serving Suggestion: Let your Grilled Lemon Herb Tofu Steaks star alongside a chorus of char-grilled veggies or a refreshing garden ensemble.

Nutritional Info: Calories: 250, Fat: 18g, Carbs: 7g, Dietary Fiber: 2g, Sugars: 1g, Protein: 16g

8. Herb-Crusted Pork Loin with Apple Chutney

(Ready in: 20 mins – plus marinating time - | Cook Duration: 45 mins | Persons: 4)

Necessary Items:

For the Pork Loin:

- Boneless pork loin (approximately 1.5 lbs or 700g): 1
- Dijon mustard: 2 tablespoons
- Minced garlic cloves: 2
- Fresh rosemary, finely chopped: 1 tablespoon
- Fresh thyme leaves: 1 tablespoon
- Salt and black pepper, to taste
- Olive oil: 2 tablespoons

For the Apple Chutney:

- Large apples, peeled, cored, and diced (sweet variety): 2
- Diced red onion: 1/2 cup
- Apple cider vinegar: 1/4 cup
- Brown sugar: 1/4 cup
- Ground cinnamon: 1/4 teaspoon
- Ground nutmeg: 1/4 teaspoon
- Salt, to taste

How to Prepare:

For the Pork Loin:

- ✓ In a small bowl, combine the Dijon mustard, minced garlic, fresh rosemary, fresh thyme, salt, and black pepper. Mix well to create the herb marinade.
- ✓ Place the pork loin in a dish and rub the herb marinade evenly over the surface of the meat. Cover and refrigerate for at least 30 minutes, or longer for more flavor (up to 24 hours).
- ✓ Preheat your oven to 350°F (175°C).
- ✓ In an ovenproof skillet or frying pan, heat the olive oil over medium-high heat. Once hot, sear the pork loin on all sides until it develops a golden crust, about 2-3 minutes per side.
- ✓ Transfer the skillet to the preheated oven and roast the pork loin for 30-35 minutes or until the internal temperature reaches 145°F (63°C). Use a meat thermometer to check the temperature.
- ✓ Once done, remove the pork loin from the oven and let it rest for about 5 minutes before slicing.

For the Apple Chutney:

- ✓ In a saucepan, combine the diced apples, diced red onion, apple cider vinegar, brown sugar, ground cinnamon, ground nutmeg, and a pinch of salt.

- ✓ Cook over medium heat, stirring occasionally, until the apples are tender and the chutney has thickened, about 15-20 minutes.

- ✓ Remove the apple chutney from heat and let it cool slightly.

To Serve:

- ✓ Slice the herb-crusted pork loin into thick slices.

- ✓ Serve the pork loin slices with a generous spoonful of apple chutney on top.

- ✓ Optionally, garnish with additional fresh herbs or a drizzle of the chutney sauce.

Nutritional Info: Calories: 350, Fat: 11g, Carb: 34g, Fiber: 3g, Sugars: 27g, Protein: 30g

9. Pomegranate Glazed Salmon with Roasted Brussels Sprouts

(Ready in: 15 min – plus marinating time - | Cook Duration: 25 min | Persons: 4)

Necessary Items:

For the Pomegranate Glazed Salmon:

- Salmon fillets (approximately 6 oz/170g each): 4
- Pomegranate juice: 1/2 cup
- Honey: 2 tablespoons
- Minced garlic cloves: 2
- Fresh thyme leaves: 1 teaspoon
- Salt and black pepper, to taste
- Olive oil: 2 tablespoons

For the Roasted Brussels Sprouts:

- Brussels sprouts (about 1 lb or 450g), trimmed and halved: 1 lb
- Olive oil: 2 tablespoons
- Salt and black pepper, to taste
- Grated Parmesan cheese (optional): 1/4 cup

How to Prepare:

For the Pomegranate Glazed Salmon:

- ✓ In a bowl, whisk together the pomegranate juice, honey, minced garlic, fresh thyme leaves, salt, and black pepper to create the glaze.

- ✓ Place the salmon fillets in a dish and pour half of the pomegranate glaze over them. Reserve the remaining glaze for later. Allow the salmon to marinate for at least 15 minutes or longer for more flavor.

- ✓ Preheat your oven to 375°F (190°C).

- ✓ In an ovenproof skillet or frying pan, heat the olive oil over medium-high heat. Once hot, add the marinated salmon fillets (skin side down, if they have skin) and sear for about 2-3 minutes until the salmon develops a golden crust.

- ✓ Transfer the skillet to the preheated oven and roast the salmon for 12-15 minutes, or until it flakes easily with a fork.

✓ While the salmon is roasting, prepare the roasted Brussels sprouts.

For the Roasted Brussels Sprouts:

✓ Toss the trimmed and halved Brussels sprouts with olive oil, salt, and black pepper in a baking dish.

✓ Roast them in the same oven as the salmon for about 20-25 minutes or until they are tender and slightly crispy on the outside.

✓ Optional: Sprinkle grated Parmesan cheese over the roasted Brussels sprouts during the last 5 minutes of roasting for added flavor.

To Serve:

✓ Place the roasted Brussels sprouts on individual plates.

✓ Top with a salmon fillet.

✓ Drizzle the reserved pomegranate glaze over the salmon.

✓ Optionally, garnish with fresh thyme leaves or pomegranate seeds for a burst of color and flavor.

Nutritional Info: Calories: 450, Fat: 20g, Carb: 32g, Fiber: 6g, Sugars: 20g, Protein: 36g

10. Mexican Cauliflower Rice Bowl

(Cook Duration: 15 minutes | Ready in: 15 minutes | Persons: 4)

Necessary Items:

For the Cauliflower Rice:

- Grated or processed cauliflower (1 large head)
- Olive oil: 1 tablespoon
- Finely chopped small onion: 1
- Minced garlic cloves: 2
- Ground cumin: 1 teaspoon
- Chili powder: 1 teaspoon
- Salt and black pepper, to taste
- Juice of 1 lime

For the Black Bean and Corn Salsa:

- Black beans, drained and rinsed (15 oz can): 1
- Corn kernels (fresh or frozen): 1 cup
- Cherry tomatoes, halved: 1 cup
- Finely chopped red onion: 1/2
- Chopped fresh cilantro: 1/4 cup
- Juice of 1 lime
- Salt and black pepper, to taste

For Toppings:

- Sliced avocado
- Greek yogurt or sour cream (optional)
- Salsa (optional)
- Fresh cilantro leaves

How to Prepare:

For the Cauliflower Rice:

- ✓ In a large skillet, heat the olive oil over medium heat. Add the chopped onion and minced garlic. Sauté for 2-3 minutes until they become fragrant and translucent.

- ✓ Add the grated or processed cauliflower to the skillet. Season with ground cumin, chili powder, salt, and black pepper. Sauté for about 5-7 minutes, stirring frequently, until the cauliflower rice is tender.

- ✓ Remove the skillet from heat, and drizzle the lime juice over the cauliflower rice. Stir to combine. Set aside.

For the Black Bean and Corn Salsa:

- ✓ In a mixing bowl, combine the black beans, corn kernels, cherry tomatoes, finely chopped red onion, and fresh cilantro.

- ✓ Drizzle the lime juice over the salsa and season with salt and black pepper. Toss to combine.

To Assemble:

- ✓ Divide the Mexican cauliflower rice among four bowls.

- ✓ Top each bowl with a generous portion of the black bean and corn salsa.

- ✓ Add sliced avocado on top of the salsa.

- ✓ Optionally, garnish with a dollop of Greek yogurt or sour cream, a spoonful of salsa, and fresh cilantro leaves.

Nutritional Info: Calories: 220, Fat: 6g, Carb: 36g. Dietary Fiber: 11g, Sugars: 6g, Protein: 9g

---

11. Spinach and Artichoke Stuffed Chicken Thighs
(Ready in: 20 minutes | Cook Duration: 30 minutes | Persons: 4)

Necessary Items:

For the Stuffed Chicken Thighs:

- Boneless, skinless chicken thighs: 4
- Fresh spinach leaves: 1 cup
- Canned artichoke hearts, drained and chopped: 1/2 cup
- Softened cream cheese: 1/2 cup
- Grated Parmesan cheese: 1/4 cup
- Minced garlic cloves: 2
- Italian seasoning: 1 teaspoon
- Salt and black pepper, to taste
- Cooking twine (optional)

For the Lemon Garlic Butter Sauce:

- Butter: 2 tablespoons
- Minced garlic cloves: 2
- Lemon juice: Juice of 1 lemon
- Lemon zest: Zest of 1 lemon

- Salt and black pepper, to taste
- Fresh parsley, chopped (optional, for garnish)

How to Prepare:

For the Stuffed Chicken Thighs:

- ✓ Stage Set-Up: Ignite the warmth in your oven's heart, setting it to a passionate 375°F (190°C).
- ✓ Enchanting Concoction: Dive into a mixing spell, swirling together spirited spinach, adventurous artichoke hearts, creamy cloud of cheese, regal Parmesan shavings, aromatic garlic whispers, and the Italian herb waltz, seasoned with salt and pepper. Make sure they dance harmoniously.
- ✓ Chicken's Solo: Display the chicken thighs like blank canvases, sprinkling both sides with a hint of salt and pepper.
- ✓ Filling the Dance Card: Share the enchanting concoction among the chicken performers, ensuring each gets an even spread of the magic.
- ✓ Curtain Roll: Envelop each thigh with its newfound magic, and if they're trying to spill their secrets, secure them with culinary threads. Place them, seam whispering downwards, on their oven stage.
- ✓ Oven's Ballet: Let them dance in the oven's embrace for a graceful 25-30 minutes or until their performance is impeccable and they reach a heartwarming 165°F (74°C).

For the Lemon Garlic Butter Sauce:

- ✓ Musical Start: In a conductor's saucepan, let butter waves flow under medium notes. Introduce garlic tunes and let them play for about 1-2 minutes, filling the air with aromatic melodies.
- ✓ Citrus Crescendo: As the notes climax, pull away from the heat and infuse zesty lemon rhythms, both juice and zest. Season it all with salt and pepper's harmony.

To Serve:

- ✓ With the chicken ballet complete, serenade them with the lemon-garlic butter symphony, letting the melodies intertwine. For a touch of encore, sprinkle a fresh parsley ovation. Now, let your taste buds applaud!

Nutritional Info: Calories: 320, Total Fat: 23g, Carb: 7g, Fiber: 2g, Sugars: 2g, Protein: 24g

12. Coconut Curry Butternut Squash Soup

(Ready in: 15 minutes | Cook Duration: 40 minutes | Persons: 4)

Necessary Items:

- Diced butternut squash (medium-sized), peeled and seeded: 1
- Coconut milk (14 ounces can): 1 can
- Olive oil: 1 tablespoon
- Chopped onion (small): 1
- Minced garlic cloves: 2
- Minced fresh ginger: 1 tablespoon
- Curry powder: 1 tablespoon
- Ground cumin: 1/2 teaspoon
- Ground coriander: 1/2 teaspoon

- Red pepper flakes (adjust to taste): 1/4 teaspoon
- Vegetable broth: 3 cups
- Salt and black pepper, to taste
- Fresh cilantro leaves for garnish (optional)

How to Prepare:

- ✓ Olive Overture: With a generous swish of olive oil, set the stage in a grand pot over a medium flame. As the spotlight warms, invite the finely-chopped onion for its solo performance, captivating the audience for a brief 2-3 minutes till it dons a sheer, glistening costume.
- ✓ Garlic & Ginger Groove: As the onion's applause lingers, welcome the spirited duo of minced garlic and zesty ginger. Their rhythmic dance, lasting 1-2 minutes, fills the air with an aromatic allure.
- ✓ Spice Serenade: Next, let the harmonious trio of curry powder, cumin, and coriander waltz in, with a pinch of red pepper flakes for flair. Their 1-minute performance, a delicate ballet, ensures the spices are toasted to perfection.
- ✓ Butternut Ballad: On cue, the butternut squash steps in, its vibrant colors dancing gracefully for another 2-3 minutes in harmony with the ensemble.
- ✓ Coconut Crescendo: Gently pour a river of creamy coconut milk followed by the soothing tones of vegetable broth. Let the ensemble rise to a thrilling boil, only to gently waltz back to a low, simmering embrace for about 30 minutes, letting the squash soften into tenderness.
- ✓ Blending Ballet: With grace and caution, blend the simmering soup into a velvety potion of warmth. Whether you choose the delicate strokes of an immersion blender or the grand spins of a regular one, remember to handle the hot melodies with care.
- ✓ Seasoned Solo: As the blended symphony returns to the pot, sprinkle the notes of salt and pepper, letting them tune the ensemble for another 5-minute performance.
- ✓ Grand Finale: Serve this velvety Butternut Bliss piping hot, and if the mood strikes, let a few fresh cilantro leaves take a bow on top.

Nutritional Info: Calories: 220, Fat: 16g, Carb: 18g, Dietary Fiber: 4g, Sugars: 3g, Protein: 2g

13. Roasted Beet and Walnut Salad with Citrus Dressing

(Ready in: 15 minutes | Cook Duration: 45 minutes | Persons: 4)

Necessary Items:

For the Roasted Beet Salad:

- Beets (4 medium-sized), washed and trimmed: 4
- Toasted and roughly chopped walnuts: 1 cup
- Mixed salad greens (6 cups, e.g., spinach, arugula, or mesclun)
- Crumbled feta cheese (optional): 1/2 cup
- Chopped fresh parsley: 2 tablespoons
- Salt and black pepper, to taste

For the Citrus Dressing:

- Juice of 1 orange
- Juice of 1 lemon
- Zest of 1 lemon
- Olive oil: 2 tablespoons
- Honey (or maple syrup for a vegan option): 1 tablespoon
- Dijon mustard: 1 teaspoon
- Minced small clove of garlic: 1
- Salt and black pepper, to taste

How to Prepare:

- ✓ Oven's Warm Welcome: Ignite your oven's spirit to a toasty 400°F (200°C).
- ✓ Beet Retreat: Lovingly swaddle each beet in a cozy aluminum foil blanket and let them lounge on a baking tray. Treat them to a 45-minute sauna session or until they yield to the gentle poke of a fork. Once cooled, unveil their vibrant beauty and fashion them into circles or elegant wedges.
- ✓ Walnut Waltz: As the beets bask, let the walnuts groove on a skillet stage over medium heat. For a five-minute fiery fiesta, keep them moving till they release their aromatic charm. Once done, let them cool off and give them a rustic chop.
- ✓ Bowl of Abundance: In a grand salad amphitheater, gather the lush greens, the roasted beet aristocrats, dancing walnuts, and, if you fancy, sprinkle in some crumbled feta confetti.
- ✓ Citrus Symphony: Conduct a melodious blend of orange and lemon tunes, invigorated with lemon zest, harmonized by olive oil, sweetened by honey, emboldened by Dijon mustard, and nuanced with whispers of garlic, salt, and pepper in a petite orchestra bowl.
- ✓ Dress to Impress: Lavishly shower the citrus serenade over the ensemble in the bowl. Gently sway the ingredients together, ensuring every morsel feels the zest.
- ✓ Finishing Flourish: Grace your creation with sprigs of fresh parsley, and if your palate desires, sprinkle a dash of salt and pepper. Present it forth as a gastronomic ballet for the senses.

Nutritional Info: Calories: 275, Fat: 19g, Carb: 23g, Fiber: 5g, Sugars: 13g, Protein: 6g

14. Lemon Rosemary Grilled Swordfish

(Ready in: 15 minutes, Cook Duration: 10-12 minutes, Persons: 4)

Necessary Items:

- Swordfish fillets (4, about 6 ounces each)
- Zest and juice of 1 lemon
- Minced garlic (2 cloves)
- Finely chopped fresh rosemary (2 tablespoons)
- Olive oil (2 tablespoons)
- Salt and black pepper, to taste
- Lemon wedges
- Fresh rosemary sprigs (optional)

How to Prepare:

- ✓ Citrus Serendipity: In your most cherished petite bowl, craft a zesty symphony using bright lemon zest, tangy lemon juice, aromatic minced garlic, fresh-cut rosemary, a drizzle of olive oil, and a dash each of salt and black pepper. This magical potion is the secret song for your swordfish!

- ✓ Swordfish Soiree: Lay your majestic swordfish fillets in a graceful dance arena, be it a dish or a zip-top bag. Pour the freshly crafted citrus song over them, ensuring every inch bathes in its melodies. Cloak the dish or seal the song within the bag and send it to the chill chambers (refrigerator) for a brief 15-minute ballad of flavors.
- ✓ Fiery Stage Prep: Fire up your grill, aiming for a passionate medium-high embrace (around 400°F or 200°C). Gently brush the grill grates with love and oil to ensure a smooth dance floor for the fish.
- ✓ Encore Entrance: Bid farewell to the marinade and gently dab the swordfish with paper towels, preparing them for their spotlight moment.
- ✓ Grill Gala: Let the swordfish groove on the grill for a captivating 5-6 minutes on each side. Their readiness is marked by easy flaking and charming grill tattoos. Remember, their dance might be shorter or longer depending on their thickness.
- ✓ Curtain Call: With grace, escort the perfectly grilled swordfish to their final resting stage, a beautiful serving platter.
- ✓ Finale Flourish: Adorn with lemony crescents and rosemary wands for an encore presentation. Serve while the applause (heat) is still high, and let the taste buds revel in the celebration!

Nutritional Info: Calories: 290, Fat: 12g, Carb: 3g, Fiber: 1g, Sugars: 0g, Protein: 42g

---

15. Moroccan Spiced Chickpea Stew
(Ready in: 15 minutes | Cook Duration: 30 minutes | Persons: 4)

Necessary Items:

- Olive oil (2 tablespoons)
- Finely chopped large onion
- Minced garlic (2 cloves)
- Diced red bell pepper
- Diced yellow bell pepper
- Ground cumin (1 teaspoon)
- Ground coriander (1 teaspoon)
- Ground paprika (1 teaspoon)
- Ground cinnamon (1/2 teaspoon)
- Cayenne pepper (1/4 teaspoon, adjust to taste)
- Chickpeas, drained and rinsed (1 can, 15 ounces)
- Diced tomatoes (1 can, 14 ounces)
- Vegetable broth (3 cups)
- Diced butternut squash (1 cup)
- Diced zucchini (1 cup)
- Salt and black pepper, to taste
- Fresh cilantro leaves (optional)
- Lemon wedges

How to Prepare:

- ✓ Onion Orchestra: In your grand culinary cauldron, serenade olive oil with warmth on a medium tune. Introduce finely diced onions to the pot and dance with them for a 3-4 minute waltz until their grace turns sheer.

- ✓ Spice Soiree: Enrich the cauldron with aromatic minced garlic, vibrant dice of red and yellow bell peppers, and a tapestry of spices: cumin's warmth, coriander's whisper, paprika's embrace, cinnamon's allure, and the playful kick of cayenne. Serenade these ingredients together for another 2-3 minutes, letting their fragrant songs meld.
- ✓ Veggie Virtuoso: Welcome aboard the hearty chickpeas, lush diced tomatoes, nourishing broth, sweet butternut chunks, and crisp zucchini dice. Season with salt and black pepper; they are creating a harmonious blend.
- ✓ Symphonic Simmer: Usher this medley to a crescendo (boil) and then, like a calming lullaby, lower the tune to a gentle simmer. Let this ensemble perform under the cauldron's lid for 20-25 minutes, letting the veggies soften in their embrace.
- ✓ Finishing Flourishes: Sample this melody and adjust the notes. Crave a spicier edge? Invite more cayenne. Need balance? Introduce salt and pepper.
- ✓ Grand Finale: Pour the Moroccan Chickpea Medley into majestic bowls. Garnish with the vibrant green of fresh cilantro and accompany with the zesty rhythm of lemon wedges, enhancing the final culinary chorus. Enjoy the feast!

Nutritional Info: Calories: 250, Fat: 7g, Carb: 41g, Fiber: 10g, Sugars: 9g, Protein: 10g

16. Creamy Pumpkin and Sage Risotto

(Ready in: 10 minutes | Cook Duration: 25 minutes | Persons: 4)

Necessary Items:

- Arborio rice (1 1/2 cups)
- Vegetable broth (4 cups)
- Canned pumpkin puree (1 cup)
- Dry white wine (optional, 1/2 cup)
- Finely chopped small onion
- Minced garlic (2 cloves)
- Olive oil (2 tablespoons)
- Fresh sage leaves, chopped (2 tablespoons)
- Grated Parmesan cheese (1/2 cup)
- Salt and black pepper, to taste
- Fresh sage leaves

How to Prepare:

- ✓ Broth Ballet: In a dancer's posture, gracefully warm your vegetable broth in a medium-sized pot. The broth should pirouette on the brink of boiling but not fully leap.
- ✓ Onion Overture: With a large skillet as your stage, caress olive oil under a medium spotlight. Introduce finely chopped onion to the stage, letting it dance for 2-3 minutes until its glow captures the audience.
- ✓ Rice Rhapsody: Amidst the onion's applause, welcome the aromatic whispers of minced garlic and the star performer Arborio rice. Engage them in a 2-3 minute duet, ensuring the rice pirouettes to a light golden hue.
- ✓ Wine Waltz: If you've chosen white wine as your guest performer, let it sweep onto the stage, mingling with the rice. This act continues till the wine's notes are a soft echo.
- ✓ Broth Ballet Act II: As if penning a poetic verse, ladle in your warm broth, one stanza at a time. Each line is absorbed, and the next begins; a continuous rhythmic dance till the rice sways creamy and al dente – an 18-20 minute performance.

- ✓ Pumpkin Pas de Deux: Introduce the smooth allure of canned pumpkin puree and the aromatic twirl of freshly chopped sage. Their dance, lasting 2-3 minutes, unites the flavors in an elegant embrace.
- ✓ Cheesy Crescendo: Off the heat, weave in the robust notes of grated Parmesan, followed by the harmonious chords of salt and black pepper.
- ✓ Grand Finale: Spotlight on! Serve this Creamy Pumpkin and Sage Risotto in beautiful bowls, crowned with fresh sage if you're feeling a touch dramatic.

Nutritional Info: Calories: 360, Fat: 9g, Carbohydrates: 60g, Fiber: 4g, Sugars: 3g, Protein: 9g

17. Pesto Spaghetti Squash with Cherry Tomatoes

(Ready in: 15 minutes | Cook Duration: 40 minutes | Persons: 4)

Necessary Items:

- Large spaghetti squash (1)
- Cherry tomatoes, halved (1 cup)
- Pesto sauce (store-bought or homemade, 1/2 cup)
- Grated Parmesan cheese (1/4 cup)
- Olive oil (2 tablespoons)
- Salt and black pepper, to taste
- Fresh basil leaves

How to Prepare:

- ✓ Squash Serenade: Set the stage by heating your oven to a cozy 375°F (190°C). Take the spaghetti squash and, with precision, slice it from top to bottom. Dive into its core and extract the seeds, setting the stage for what's to come.
- ✓ Olive Oil Overture: Paint each half of the squash with a golden olive oil glaze, sprinkling a pinch of salt and pepper for that added zest.
- ✓ Baking Ballet: On a parchment-papered dance floor (baking sheet), let the squash halves lay face down, ready to waltz in the oven's warmth. Allow a 30-40 minute performance until the inside twirls with the light touch of a fork.
- ✓ Tomato Tango: While our main dancer is on stage, choreograph the cherry tomatoes. Split them gracefully into pairs and keep them waiting in the wings.
- ✓ Strand Symphony: Once our star, the squash, has finished its act, let it rest, gathering its energy. Then, with the baton (fork) in hand, orchestrate the strands, producing spaghetti-like melodies.
- ✓ Sauté Soirée: In the grand skillet arena, let a splash of olive oil set the mood. The cherry tomato duos make their entrance, swaying for a short 2-3 minute number until they soften with grace.
- ✓ Pesto Performance: Introduce the spaghetti squash strands back into the mix, harmonizing with the tomatoes. Now, let the pesto take center stage, swirling and merging for another 2-3 minutes, infusing its flavors.
- ✓ Cheese Chorus: As the curtain prepares to fall, shower the ensemble with the rich notes of grated Parmesan cheese, stirring them into a delicious crescendo.
- ✓ Final Flourish: Present this masterpiece in bowls, and if you're in the mood, let a few fresh basil leaves take a bow on top

Nutritional Info: Calories: 280, Fat: 20, Carbohydrates: 23g, Fiber: 5g, Sugars: 7g, Protein: 6g

18. Walnut-Crusted Turkey Cutlets

(Ready in: 15 minutes | Cook Duration: 15 minutes | Persons: 4)

Necessary Items:

- Turkey cutlets (4, about 1 pound)
- Finely chopped walnuts (1 cup)
- Whole wheat breadcrumbs (1/2 cup)
- Grated Parmesan cheese (1/4 cup)
- Chopped fresh parsley (2 tablespoons)
- Dried thyme (1 teaspoon)
- Eggs (2)
- Olive oil (2 tablespoons)
- Salt and black pepper, to taste

For Serving (optional):

- Lemon wedges

How to Prepare:

- ✓ Nutty Ensemble Preparation: In a dish that's just the right depth, summon walnuts, breadcrumbs, the majestic Parmesan, vibrant parsley, and the ever-so-aromatic dried thyme. Add a touch of salt and pepper for a little extra zing, then blend them into a harmonious mix.
- ✓ Egg Euphoria: In a neighboring dish, create a pool of whipped dreams by beating the eggs into submission.
- ✓ Turkey Tantalization: Season those turkey cutlets! A sprinkle of salt and pepper does wonders for their personality.
- ✓ Double-dip Delight: Take each turkey artist and dip them into our egg whirlpool, ensuring they are glistening from edge to edge. Without hesitation, introduce them to the nutty ensemble, ensuring they wear their walnut wardrobe with pride.
- ✓ Sizzling Soiree: Set the stage with olive oil in a skillet over medium-high fire. Await its beckoning call - that shimmer that says, "It's showtime."
- ✓ Golden Performance: With grace, lay each walnut-adorned turkey cutlet on the stage. Let them dance for about 3-4 minutes on each side, aiming for a finale of golden brown perfection.
- ✓ Curtain Call: Once their performance ends, escort the turkey stars onto a paper towel carpet to bask, ensuring they retain only the good kind of oils.
- ✓ Encore Presentation: Serve these Walnut Wonders steaming and, for an added flourish, let lemon wedges grace their side.

Nutritional Info: Calories: 380, Fat: 24g, Carb: 10g, Fiber: 2g, Sugars: 1g, Protein: 33g

19. Sesame-Ginger Salmon with Bok Choy

(Ready in: 15 minutes, Cook Duration: 15 minutes, Persons: 4)

Necessary Items:

- Salmon fillets (4, about 6 ounces each)
- Baby bok choy (4, halved lengthwise)
- Sesame oil (2 tablespoons)
- Low-sodium soy sauce (2 tablespoons)

- Rice vinegar (2 tablespoons)
- Minced fresh ginger (1 tablespoon)
- Minced garlic cloves (2)
- Honey (1 tablespoon)
- Sesame seeds (1 tablespoon)
- Salt and black pepper, to taste

For Garnish (optional):

- Sliced green onions

How to Prepare:

- ✓ Warm Welcome: Ignite your oven's passion and set its heart to a balmy 400°F (200°C).
- ✓ Magic Potion Prep: In an enchanting vessel, summon the powers of sesame oil, whispering soy sauce, vibrant rice vinegar, the zesty spirit of ginger and garlic, sweet honey, and loyal sesame seeds. Swirl them into an elixir with the whisk of destiny.
- ✓ Salmon's Spa Day: Lay your salmon stars in a lounging dish, pampering them with half of the magic potion. Let them soak in this luxury for a brief 10 minutes, remembering to flip them for an even tan.
- ✓ Bok Choy's Star Moment: As the salmon basks, ready the bok choy for their spotlight. Let these green beauties grace a baking stage, showing off their cut side. Shower them with the remaining magic potion for the perfect sheen.
- ✓ Season's Greetings: Whisper wishes of salt and pepper onto both the salmon and bok choy, ensuring these simple joys touch them.
- ✓ Duet Performance: Let the salmon and bok choy harmonize in the oven's embrace for 12-15 minutes. Await the tender notes of the bok choy and the gentle flake of the salmon as signs of a show well done.
- ✓ Grand Finale: Upon their encore exit from the oven, plate up this Sesame-Ginger duet while the applause (aromas) fill the room.
- ✓ Curtain Call: Adorn this performance with the graceful dance of green onions if the heart so desires.

Nutritional Info: Calories: 320, Fat: 17g, Carb: 11g, Fiber: 2g, Sugars: 6g, Protein: 30g

20. Cabbage Rolls with Ground Turkey and Rice

(Ready in: 30 minutes, Cook Duration: 1h, Persons: 4)

Necessary Items:

- 1 head of cabbage
- Ground turkey: 1 pound
- Cooked white rice: 1 cup
- Small onion, finely chopped: 1
- Garlic cloves, minced: 2
- Diced tomatoes (14 ounces can): 1 can
- Egg: 1
- Milk: 1/4 cup
- Dried oregano: 1 teaspoon
- Dried basil: 1 teaspoon
- Salt and black pepper, to taste
- Tomato sauce: 2 cups
- Chicken or vegetable broth: 1/2 cup
- Chopped fresh parsley for garnish (optional)

How to Prepare:

- ✓ Oven's Warm Embrace: Get your oven in the mood for magic at a cozy 350°F (175°C).
- ✓ Cabbage Spa: In a pot large enough for a royal bath, bring water to a dance. Gently whisk 12 regal cabbage leaves into the bubbling waters, letting them waltz for 3-5 minutes until they sway with ease. Lift them out, letting them cool in the breezy air.
- ✓ Turkey Tango: On the dance floor of a skillet, whirl the ground turkey around over medium beats. Break its dance moves with a spoon until it's uniformly bronzed. Cast away any excess backstage oil.
- ✓ Cast Party: Bring all-stars into the grand mixing hall - the golden turkey, fluffy white rice, ever-crunchy onion, aromatic garlic, juicy diced tomatoes, the loyal egg, creamy milk, the herbs of oregano and basil, and a sprinkle of salt and pepper. Let them dance in harmony.
- ✓ Rolling the Red Carpet: Lay a cabbage leaf like a scroll. Crown its center with the star-studded turkey and rice ensemble. Fold it into a regal robe, ensuring the ends are neatly tucked. Encore with the remaining stars.
- ✓ Saucy Interlude: In the potion bowl, blend the beautiful tomato sauce with the mysterious broth of chicken or vegetables.
- ✓ Staging the Performance: On the stage of a baking dish lay a thin red carpet of the saucy interlude. Set the cabbage royalty, seam-side down, in stately rows.
- ✓ Royal Drapery: Cascade the remaining saucy potion over our cabbage cast, ensuring they're robed in flavors.
- ✓ Oven's Curtain Call: Shield our stars with a silver foil curtain and let them perform in the oven's warmth for 45-50 minutes. Their performance peak is when the cabbage is soft, and they're bursting with flavors.
- ✓ Final Flourish: Bestow a green rain of fresh parsley for the perfect curtain call.
- ✓ Standing Ovation: Present the Turkey & Rice Cabbage Hug Rolls while they're hot, with an encore of the saucy melody.

Nutritional Info: Calories: 350, Fat: 11g, Carb: 39g, Fiber: 7g, Sugars: 10g, Protein: 26g

Chapter 7: Snack & Dessert Recipes For Intermittent Fasting

1. Coconut Chia Pudding with Mango

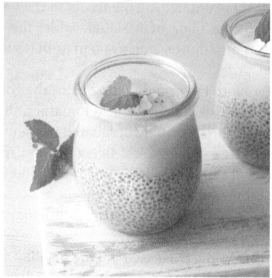

(Ready in: 10mins | Persons: 2)

Necessary Items:

- Chia seeds: 1/4 cup
- Coconut milk: 1 cup
- Honey or maple syrup (optional, for sweetness): 1 tablespoon
- Vanilla extract: 1/2 teaspoon
- Ripe mango, diced: 1
- Fresh mint leaves for garnish (optional)

How to Prepare:

✓ Elixir Beginnings: Dive into a bowl and conjure up a tropical potion by mingling chia seeds, the embrace of coconut milk, nature's sweet drizzle (honey or maple syrup), and a whisper of vanilla. Stir this magic until the chia seeds dance in unison.

✓ Rest & Settle: Let this concoction dream for a mere 5 minutes, but disturb its slumber after the first minute for a quick swirl, ensuring no chia seed feels left out.

✓ Magic Sleep: Cloak the bowl and let it slumber in the icy chambers of your fridge. Let the dreams last for 2 hours or a night-long voyage. In this time, the chia seeds will sip on the elixir and morph into a pudding sorcery.

✓ Mango's Waltz: As the grand serving moment approaches, court a ripe mango into surrendering its golden cubes.

✓ Awaken the Sorcery: Gently awaken your chilled chia creation, giving it a hearty stir. If it's too lost in its dreams, a splash more of coconut milk will bring it back to reality.

✓ Royal Presentation: Pour the chia enchantment into regal glasses or bowls, ready for the feast.

✓ Mango Coronation: Crown each serving with the golden mango treasures.

✓ Mint's Blessing: For an added touch of magic, let fresh mint leaves sprinkle their blessings. Revel in this chilled tropical delight!

Nutritional Info: Calories: 235 kcal, Carbohydrates: 24g, Fiber: 9g, Sugars: 10g, Protein: 5g, Fat: 15g, Saturated Fat: 11g, Cholesterol: 0mg, Sodium: 14mg

2. Almond and Date Energy Bites

(Ready in: 15 minutes | Persons: 12-15 bites)

Necessary Items:

- Pitted dates: 1 cup
- Almonds: 1 cup
- Unsweetened cocoa powder: 1/4 cup
- Almond butter: 1/4 cup
- Vanilla extract: 1 teaspoon
- A pinch of salt
- Shredded coconut (optional, for coating): 2 tablespoons

How to Prepare:

✓ Commence the Ritual: Into the sacred chamber of a food processor, summon the soulful dates, spirited almonds, mysterious cocoa dust, essence of almond elixir, a whiff of ethereal vanilla, and a spellbinding dash of salt.

✓ Conjure the Fusion: Awaken the spirits by sending pulses of energy, weaving them into an arcane, sticky tapestry. This act of alchemy might test your patience, so let the energies dance until they find their harmony.

✓ Elemental Adjustments: Should you discover that the mystical blend yearns for moisture, bestow upon it a touch more almond potion or whispering droplets of the elixir of life (water).

✓ Crafting the Orbs: With the grace of an ancient alchemist, reach into the blend and mold ethereal spheres that contain the power of the cosmos. The size of these energy orbs is a reflection of your intent; choose wisely.

✓ Baptism by Coconut: If the stars align, roll these precious globes in the embrace of shredded coconut, gifting them an external armor of delight.

✓ Lunar Chill Ritual: Let these orbs bask under the cool embrace of the moon (or your fridge) for a half-turn of the hourglass, solidifying their essence.

✓ Sacred Storage: Post their celestial rendezvous, nestle the Almond & Date Energy Spheres in a sanctuary (an airtight container), and let them repose in the refrigerator's embrace.

Nutritional Info: Calories: 96 kcal, Carbohydrates: 11g, Fiber: 2g, Sugars: 7g, Protein: 3g, Fat: 6g, Saturated Fat: 0.5g, Cholesterol: 0mg, Sodium: 1mg

3. Nutty Trail Mix

(Ready in: 5 minutes | Persons: 6)

Necessary Items:

- Unsalted mixed nuts (almonds, cashews, walnuts, etc.): 1 cup
- Dried cranberries or raisins: 1/2 cup
- Dark chocolate chips or chunks: 1/2 cup

- Pumpkin seeds (pepitas): 1/2 cup
- Sea salt (adjust to taste): 1/4 teaspoon
- Shredded coconut (optional): 1/4 cup

How to Prepare:

- ✓ Gathering of the Clan: In the grand arena of a mixing bowl, summon forth the valiant mixed nuts, the ruby-red dried cranberries (or their raisin counterparts), the intoxicating dark chocolate emissaries (be it chips or formidable chunks), the proud pumpkin seed warriors, and, if your journey wishes, the wispy whispers of shredded coconut.
- ✓ Awakening the Flavor Dragon: Bestow upon this gathering a gentle shower of sea salt, a mineral known to rouse the dormant spirits of flavors. Remember, in this realm, the dragon's power (saltiness) is in your hands.
- ✓ The Grand Jamboree: With grace, usher a grand dance, swirling and twirling every participant until they find their rhythm and merge into one harmonious ensemble.
- ✓ The Invitation to Distant Allies: Hear the call of exotic adventurers? Welcome them! Be it the sun-kissed dried apricots, crunchy banana heralds, or any nutty knight or seeded squire you fancy.
- ✓ The Final Resting Chamber: Lead this majestic congregation to their new dominion - airtight fortresses for extended vacations or petite sachets for those swift escapades.
- ✓ Preservation Ritual: Bestow this mix the privilege of resting in a sanctuary of cool and dry, or grant them the chill of the ice caverns (refrigerator) if that's the journey you wish for them.

Nutritional Info: Calories: 280 kcal, Carbohydrates: 23g, Fiber: 4g, Sugars: 14g, Protein: 7g, Fat: 19g, Saturated Fat: 6g, Cholesterol: 0mg, Sodium: 50mg

---

4. Cucumber Dill Greek Yogurt Dip

(Ready in: 10 minutes | Persons: 6)

Necessary Items:

- Greek yogurt: 1 cup
- Fresh lemon juice: 1 tablespoon
- Cucumber, finely grated and drained: 1/2
- Lemon zest: 1/2 teaspoon
- Fresh dill, chopped: 1 tablespoon
- Salt and black pepper, to taste
- Garlic clove, minced: 1

How to Prepare:

- ✓ Cucumber Chronicles: Embark on your journey with the humble cucumber. Unleash your skills with a trusty box grater or the magic of a food processor, turning that cucumber into delicate wisps. Once transformed, place your cucumber strands upon a mesh throne above a bowl, letting its watery tears drip away.
- ✓ A concoction of the Elders: In a mystical mixing cauldron, summon the creamy Greek yogurt, the now-tamed cucumber shreds, the fragrant whispers of fresh dill, the zesty incantations of garlic, and the spirited splashes of lemon, both its juice and zesty shavings.

- ✓ The Grand Stirring: With a motion as ancient as time, intertwine these elements, binding them together in harmony.
- ✓ Tales of Taste: Approach the potion cautiously, seasoning it with salt and pepper's elemental crystals. Yet remember, the cucumber is a siren that sometimes carries the sea's saltiness; hence, bestow salt with wisdom.
- ✓ Tuning the Elixir: Sip and savor. Does it need the playful laughter of more dill or perhaps the tangy tales of more lemon? Trust your senses.
- ✓ The Presentation Ritual: With reverence, transfer this divine concoction to its final resting place, a bowl worthy of its grandeur.
- ✓ The Final Flourish: Anoint your potion with a dill crown or perhaps a liquid gold drizzle of olive oil, symbolizing its elevation to perfection.
- ✓ Feast of the Fae: Present this elixir with nature's finest - crunchy veggies, ethereal pita chips, or wise whole-grain sentinels. Dive in, and let the enchantment begin!

Nutritional Info: Calories: 30 kcal, Carbohydrates: 2g, Protein: 3g, Fat: 1g, Saturated Fat: 0g, Cholesterol: 0mg, Sodium: 10mg, Fiber: 0g, Sugars: 1g

5. Baked Pear with Honey and Walnuts

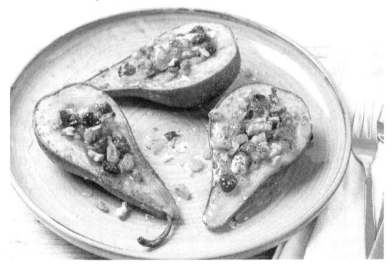

(Ready in: 10 minutes | Cook Duration: 25 minutes | Persons: 2)

Necessary Items:

- 2 ripe pears
- 2 tablespoons honey
- Chopped walnuts: 1/4 cup
- Ground cinnamon: 1/2 teaspoon
- A pinch of nutmeg (optional)
- Greek yogurt or vanilla ice cream for serving (optional)

How to Prepare:

- ✓ Prologue: Set the stage by warming the grand oven chamber to a cozy 350°F (175°C).
- ✓ Pear Spa Day: Bless the pears with a rejuvenating bath. Then, with the precision of a master sculptor, slice these beauties in half and, using a magic spoon, fashion a quaint hollow in their center, banishing any unwanted seeds.

- ✓ The Enchanted Elixir: In the goblet of dreams (or just a small bowl), conjure a potion of sweet honey, valiant walnuts, the mystique of cinnamon, and, if the stars so align, a whisper of nutmeg.
- ✓ Pear Ballroom Dance: Elegantly arrange the pears, cut side facing the sky, on their grand stage - a baking sheet or an ovenproof platter.
- ✓ Blessings from Above: Shower each pear with the ambrosial nectar, filling their hollow hearts with this golden treasure.
- ✓ Veil of Protection: Shield these royal fruits with a silvery foil canopy, ensuring they're free to transform without sticking to their protective cover.
- ✓ A Dance in the Oven: Let the pears waltz in the heated embrace of the oven for a dance that lasts about 20-25 minutes. Their readiness is heralded by a tender yield to a gentle fork prod. Remember, the nature of their dance might vary based on how ripe they came into the ballroom.
- ✓ Cooling Waltz: After their heated performance, grant them a brief respite to cool and gather their thoughts.
- ✓ The Grand Finale: Present the baked pear royalty in their full splendor. Adorn them further with a cloud of Greek yogurt or perhaps a throne of vanilla ice cream.
- ✓ Final Touches: For those who desire that extra dash of magic, sprinkle them with chopped walnut jewels or a drizzle of honey's golden kiss.

Nutritional Info: Calories: 192 kcal, Carbohydrates: 35g, Protein: 2g, Fat: 7g, Saturated Fat: 0.5g, Cholesterol: 0mg, Sodium: 1mg, Fiber: 6g, Sugars: 24g

6. Zucchini Chocolate Chip Muffins

(Ready in: 15 minutes | Cook Duration: 20-25 minutes | Persons: 12)

Necessary Items:

- All-purpose flour: 1 1/2 cups
- Whole wheat flour: 1/2 cup
- Granulated sugar: 1/2 cup
- Brown sugar, packed: 1/2 cup
- Baking powder: 1 1/2 teaspoons
- Baking soda: 1/2 teaspoon
- Salt: 1/2 teaspoon
- Ground cinnamon: 1 teaspoon
- Ground nutmeg: 1/4 teaspoon
- Large eggs: 2
- Unsalted butter, melted and cooled: 1/2 cup
- Plain Greek yogurt: 1/4 cup
- Vanilla extract: 1 teaspoon
- Grated zucchini (about 2 medium zucchinis): 1 1/2 cups
- Semi-sweet chocolate chips: 3/4 cup

How to Prepare:

- ✓ Intro to Baking: Warm your magical baking cavern (aka oven) to a toasty 350°F (175°C). While it's heating, prepare your muffin knight's armor with paper shields or give them a slick greasing.

- ✓ Alchemy in Progress: In the cauldron of creation (that's a large mixing bowl for the uninitiated), weave together the all-purpose flour, its wholesome cousin - whole wheat flour, the twin sugars (granulated and brown), baking guardians (baking powder and baking soda), a pinch of salt, and spices that whisper tales of the Orient - cinnamon and nutmeg. Stir the enchanted mixture till it sings!
- ✓ Potion of Liveliness: In a separate sacred bowl, dance the eggs into a frenzy. To this lively mix, introduce the cool, melted butter, Greek yogurt, and the essence of vanilla, blending till it resembles a potion smooth and fine.
- ✓ Confluence of Worlds: Marry the wet potion with the alchemical dry blend. Stir with reverence till they become one, but be wary of over-stirring lest the spell breaks. This union will be thick, like tales of yore.
- ✓ Zucchini's Entry: Whisper the grated zucchini to join the mix, ensuring it mingles well and loses itself in the batter's embrace.
- ✓ Chocolate's Surprise: As the final flourish, summon the semi-sweet chocolate chips, gently folding them in, letting them hide within the batter-like treasures waiting to be discovered.
- ✓ Quest Begins: Entrust each knight's armor with this special mix, filling them to a 2/3 promise of adventure.
- ✓ Baking Chronicles: Send them on a quest in your preheated oven for 20-25 minutes. The toothpick oracle marks their readiness - if it emerges clean or with tiny badges of honor (moist crumbs), the quest is complete.
- ✓ Rest and Revel: On returning from their oven journey, let them bask in their tin abode for a short 5-minute tale before setting them on a wire rack to narrate stories of their adventures.
- ✓ The Grand Feast: Once their tales are told and they've cooled, the Zucchini Chocolate Chip Muffins are ready to be devoured, promising a bite of mystery, magic, and a hint of indulgence.

Nutritional Info: Calories: 255 kcal, Carbohydrates: 38g, Protein: 4g, Fat: 11g, Saturated Fat: 7g, Cholesterol: 45mg, Sodium: 246mg, Fiber: 2g, Sugars: 21g

7. Roasted Almonds with Rosemary

(Ready in: 5 minutes | Freeze Time: 15 minutes | Persons: 4)

Necessary Items:

- Whole almonds: 2 cups
- Fresh rosemary leaves, chopped: 2 tablespoons
- Olive oil: 2 tablespoons
- Salt: 1 teaspoon
- Black pepper: 1/2 teaspoon
- Red pepper flakes (optional for a bit of heat): 1/4 teaspoon

How to Prepare:

- ✓ The Grand Stage Setup: Warm up your oven's theater to a cozy 325°F (163°C). While it's getting ready, deck out your baking stage with a silky parchment paper sheet.

- ✓ Gathering of the Ensemble: In the green room (a mixing bowl), summon the starring almonds and introduce them to the aromatic rosemary, the slick olive oil, classic salt, dashing black pepper, and, for those who like a spicy twist, the fiery red pepper flakes. Ensure the almonds waltz gracefully with these partners, getting dressed uniformly in the seasoning.
- ✓ Curtain Raiser: Lay out this seasoned cast in a choreographed single line upon the prepared baking stage.
- ✓ The Act: Let them perform their tantalizing dance in your preheated oven for 15 minutes. Peek occasionally and let them change positions once or twice for a synchronized performance. Beware! Almonds can sometimes get a little too lost in their act and char; make sure they stay on cue.
- ✓ Encore Performance: Once they've reached the peak of their golden performance and are filling the air with their alluring aroma, it's the curtain call. Gracefully escort them out, ensuring they don't overstay and turn bitter.
- ✓ Post-Show Tranquility: Let our performers rest and cool on their stage. As they regain composure, you'll notice their texture turning irresistibly crunchy.
- ✓ Applause and Delight: Once their encore is done, usher the "Roasted Almonds with Rosemary" into their green room (an airtight container) or present them center stage in a bowl to a raving audience of snack enthusiasts.

Nutritional Info: Calories: 297 kcal, Carbohydrates: 9g, Protein: 9g, Fat: 26g, Saturated Fat: 2g, Cholesterol: 0mg, Sodium: 586mg, Fiber: 5g, Sugars: 1g

---

8. Chocolate Avocado Pudding

(Persons: 4 | Ready in: 10 minutes)

Necessary Items:

- Ripe avocados, peeled and pitted: 2
- Unsweetened cocoa powder: 1/4 cup
- Honey or maple syrup (adjust to taste): 1/4 cup
- Milk (dairy or non-dairy): 1/4 cup
- Vanilla extract: 1 teaspoon
- A pinch of salt
- Optional toppings: sliced strawberries, raspberries, chopped nuts, or whipped cream

How to Prepare:

- ✓ In a food processor or blender, combine the ripe avocados, unsweetened cocoa powder, honey or maple syrup, milk, vanilla extract, and a pinch of salt.
- ✓ Blend all the ingredients until smooth and creamy. You may need to scrape down the sides of the blender or food processor and blend again to ensure there are no avocado chunks.
- ✓ Taste the pudding and adjust the sweetness if needed by adding more honey or maple syrup.
- ✓ Once the mixture is smooth and sweetened to your liking, divide it into four serving cups or bowls.

- ✓ Refrigerate the Chocolate Avocado Pudding for at least 30 minutes to chill and firm up.
- ✓ Before serving, you can add your choice of toppings such as sliced strawberries, raspberries, chopped nuts, or a dollop of whipped cream.

Nutritional Info: Calories: 237 kcal, Carbohydrates: 27g, Protein: 3g, Fat: 16g, Saturated Fat: 3g, Cholesterol: 0mg, Sodium: 37mg, Fiber: 7g, Sugars: 17g

9. Chia Seed and Berry Smoothie

(Persons: 2 | Ready in: 5 minutes)

Necessary Items:

- Mixed berries (strawberries, blueberries, raspberries): 2 cups
- Ripe banana: 1
- Chia seeds: 2 tablespoons
- Greek yogurt (or dairy-free yogurt for a vegan option): 1 cup
- Unsweetened almond milk (or any preferred milk): 1 cup
- Honey or maple syrup (optional, for sweetness): 1 tablespoon
- Ice cubes (optional)
- Fresh berries and mint leaves for garnish (optional)

How to Prepare:

- ✓ Opening Act: Assemble our main performers – vibrant mixed berries, the ever-smooth banana, mysterious chia seeds, creamy Greek yogurt, silky almond milk, and a touch of honey (for those who like the Dance a tad sweeter) – on the blender stage.
- ✓ Twist in the Tale: For a frosty grand finale and a luxurious thickness to our ballet, introduce a few ice cube dancers to the mix.
- ✓ The Dance Begins: Engage in a blending waltz, ensuring every element intertwines harmoniously. Should our ballet troupe feel too packed on stage, invite a splash more of almond milk to free up their moves.
- ✓ Intermission: Pause and take a sip. The ballet should be sweet but not overpowering. If the Dance lacks sweetness, a drizzle of honey or maple syrup can adjust the tempo.
- ✓ Grand Finale: With the performance reaching its crescendo, let the Berry Bliss Ballet cascade gracefully into two opulent glasses.
- ✓ Encore: For an encore bursting with color and zest, shower the top with a few fresh berries and mint leaves.

Nutritional Info: Calories: 237 kcal, Carbohydrates: 44g, Protein: 8g, Fat: 6g, Saturated Fat: 1g, Cholesterol: 6mg, Sodium: 82mg, Fiber: 10g, Sugars: 26g

10. Cranberry and Almond Rice Cakes

(Persons: 2 | Ready in: 10 minutes)

Necessary Items:

- Plain or whole-grain rice cakes: 4
- Almond butter: 2 tablespoons
- Dried cranberries: 1/4 cup
- Sliced almonds: 2 tablespoons

- Honey or maple syrup for drizzling (optional)
- Fresh mint leaves for garnish (optional)

How to Prepare:

- ✓ Lay out the rice cakes on a clean serving platter or individual plates.
- ✓ Spread a generous layer of almond butter on each rice cake.
- ✓ Sprinkle dried cranberries evenly over the almond butter-covered rice cakes.
- ✓ Next, sprinkle the sliced almonds on top of the cranberries.
- ✓ If you prefer a touch of sweetness, drizzle honey or maple syrup over the rice cakes.
- ✓ Optionally, garnish with a few fresh mint leaves to add a burst of color and freshnes

Nutritional Info: Calories: 252 kcal, Carbohydrates: 35g, Protein: 6g, Fat: 11g, Saturated Fat: 1g, Cholesterol: 0mg, Sodium: 14mg, Fiber: 2g, Sugars: 13g

11. Cinnamon Raisin Rice Pudding

(Persons: 4 | Ready in: 10 minutes | Cook Duration: 30 minutes)

Necessary Items:

- Arborio rice (or short-grain rice): 1 cup
- Raisins: 1/2 cup
- Milk (whole or 2%): 4 cups
- Vanilla extract: 1 teaspoon
- Granulated sugar: 1/2 cup
- Pinch of salt
- Ground cinnamon: 1/2 teaspoon
- Ground cinnamon and raisins for garnish (optional)

How to Prepare:

- ✓ Setting Sail: In your trusty saucepan vessel, welcome aboard the rice and its first milk crew of 2 cups. Embark on a medium-heat journey until the seas begin to boil gently, stirring the waters frequently to keep peace among the crew.
- ✓ Navigating Calmer Seas: As the rice claims the milky ocean, dial down the heat to a serene simmer. Gradually, like waves kissing the shore, introduce the remaining milk in about 1/2 cup intervals, ensuring the seas are well-navigated with a stir.
- ✓ The Sweetness Storm: As you sail, sprinkle in the treasures of sugar, cinnamon whispers, and a hint of salty breeze. Continue your voyage, stirring and simmering until the rice feels like soft clouds and the milky ocean thickens, typically around a 25-30 minute mark.
- ✓ Docking at Pudding Land: Upon reaching the creamy shores of Pudding Land, pull your saucepan vessel off the heat. Invite the raisins on board and whisper in the vanilla tales. If you hear the calls for more cinnamon tales, sprinkle as desired.
- ✓ Rest & Revel: Allow your creamy creation to rest, embracing the Pudding Land's breeze for a few moments. If the pudding feels too settled, a splash of milk can bring back its lively spirit.

- ✓ Feasting under the Cinnamon Stars: Serve your Cinnamon Raisin Rice Pudding under a blanket of warm comfort or the chill of night—shower with cinnamon stardust and a few more raisin companions for an epic tale on every plate.

Nutritional Info: Calories: 380 kcal, Carbohydrates: 74g, Protein: 8g, Fat: 6g, Saturated Fat: 3g, Cholesterol: 15mg, Sodium: 115mg, Fiber: 1g, Sugars: 43g

12. Apple Cinnamon Oatmeal Cookies

(Persons: 24 cookies| Ready in: 15 minutes | Cook Duration: 1215mins)

Necessary Items:

- Old-fashioned oats: 1 1/2 cups
- All-purpose flour: 1 cup
- Baking soda: 1/2 teaspoon
- Ground cinnamon: 1/2 teaspoon
- Salt: 1/4 teaspoon
- Unsalted butter, softened: 1/2 cup
- Granulated sugar: 1/2 cup
- Brown sugar, packed: 1/2 cup
- Large egg: 1
- Pure vanilla extract: 1 teaspoon
- Peeled, cored, and finely diced apple (about 1 medium-sized apple): 1 cup
- Chopped walnuts (optional): 1/2 cup

How to Prepare:

- ✓ Sunrise Over the Oven Kingdom: Ignite the fires of your oven kingdom, warming it to 350°F (175°C). Adorn your baking terrains with the magical parchment scrolls or the shields of silicone.
- ✓ Conjuring the Earthy Potion: In a mystical medium bowl, whisper to the oats, summon the flour, sprinkle the baking soda, call forth the ground cinnamon, and invoke the salt. Let them mingle and dance together. Set this potion aside for the next ritual.
- ✓ Chant of the Buttery Clouds: In the grand ceremonial bowl, perform the sacred dance by swirling the softened butter, granulated sugar, and brown sugar. Beat until they transform into creamy clouds, radiating sweetness.
- ✓ The Elixir of Life: Introduce the soul of an egg and the essence of vanilla to your buttery clouds. Continue the rhythmic beat, making sure they become one with the universe.
- ✓ Union of the Earth and Sky: Slowly merge the Earthy Potion with the Buttery Clouds, ensuring that the elements embrace each other in harmony.
- ✓ Gifts from the Enchanted Orchard: With grace and care, fold in the blessings of the diced apple and the sacred pieces of walnut (if chosen from the pantry of wonders).
- ✓ Moonlit Drops on Starry Plains: With the hands blessed by cookie spirits, drop moonlit dollops of the enchanted dough onto your prepared terrains, ensuring they have room to dance about 2 inches apart.
- ✓ Golden Embrace of the Oven Kingdom: Let your moonlit dollops be caressed by the warm embrace of the oven for 12-15 minutes. Their edges will shimmer golden, signaling their transformation.

- ✓ Rest Under the Shade of the Cooling Trees: Once emerged from the oven, let the cookie spirits rest under the cooling trees on the terrain for a few moments. Then, let them soar to wire forests to cool under the twinkling stars.
- ✓ Sleep in the Enchanted Box: As they dream of sweet adventures, nestle your Apple Cinnamon Oatmeal Cookie spirits in the enchanted airtight chests, preserving their magic till the next feast.

Nutritional Info: Calories: 125 kcal, Carbohydrates: 17g, Protein: 2g, Fat: 6g, Saturated Fat: 3g, Cholesterol: 18mg, Sodium: 52mg, Fiber: 1g, Sugars: 9g

13. Raspberry Almond Thumbprint Cookies

(Persons: 12 | Ready in: 15 minutes | Cook Duration: 12 minutes)

Necessary Items:

- Almond flour: 1 cup
- Coconut oil, softened: 1/4 cup
- Maple syrup or honey: 2 tablespoons

- Almond extract: 1/2 teaspoon
- Raspberry jam (no added sugar): 1/4 cup

How to Prepare:

- ✓ The Curtain Rises: Kindle the warmth of your oven stage to 350°F (175°C) and drape the baking sheet with a parchment paper ballet stage floor.
- ✓ The Dancer's Prelude: In the backstage dressing bowl, choreograph almond flour, melted coconut oil ballet shoes, the sweet nectar of maple (or honey), and the soulful essence of almond into a harmonious dance routine, creating a malleable dough ensemble.
- ✓ Audition for the Lead: Take the spotlight with about 1 tablespoon of dough, twirling it gracefully into a ballerina form. Position these lead dancers gracefully onto the waiting stage.
- ✓ The Dramatic Pause: With the gentle poise of a thumb, make a heartfelt gesture, pressing a little stage center on each ballerina cookie, setting the stage for the star of the show.
- ✓ Raspberry's Solo: Into this stage center, pour the passionate raspberry jam, letting it shine and take center stage.
- ✓ The Grand Performance: As the audience (oven) watches in anticipation, let the cookie ballerinas dazzle and dance for about 12 minutes, or until their edges blush a golden brown hue.
- ✓ Curtain Call: Once the performance reaches its breathtaking finale, let the dancers rest on the stage, catching their breath for a few moments, before whisking them away to the cooling balconies (wire racks) to refresh and rejuvenate.
- ✓ Encore in the Velvet Box: Admire and preserve the beauty of your Raspberry Almond Thumbprint Ballerinas in an airtight velvet box, letting them stay at room temperature, ready for their next performance for up to 5 mesmerizing days.

Nutritional Info: Calories: 110kcal | Fat: 8g | Carb: 8g | Fiber: 2g | Sugar: 4g | Protein: 2g

14. No-Bake Oatmeal Energy Bars

(Persons: 12 | Ready in: 15 minutes | Cook Duration: 1h)

Necessary Items:

- Rolled oats: 1 cup
- Almond butter: 1/2 cup
- Honey or maple syrup: 1/4 cup
- Unsweetened shredded coconut: 1/4 cup
- Chopped almonds: 1/4 cup
- Dried cranberries or other dried fruits: 1/4 cup

How to Prepare:

- ✓ In a large mixing bowl, combine rolled oats, almond butter, honey (or maple syrup), shredded coconut, chopped almonds, and dried cranberries.
- ✓ Mix well until all the ingredients are evenly distributed and the mixture sticks together when pressed.
- ✓ Line a baking dish with parchment paper.
- ✓ Press the oat mixture into the baking dish, smoothing the top with a spatula or your hands.
- ✓ Refrigerate for at least 1 hour to firm up before cutting into bars.
- ✓ Cut into bars or squares and serve.
- ✓ Store the oatmeal energy bars in an airtight container in the refrigerator for up to 1 week.

Nutritional Info: Calories: 170kcal | Fat: 10g | Carb: 17g | Fiber: 3g | Sugar: 8g | Protein: 4g

15. Lemon Sorbet with Mint

(Persons: 4 | Ready in: 15 minutes | Freezing Time: 4-6 hours)

Necessary Items:

- Fresh lemon juice (from about 6 lemons): 1 cup
- Water: 1 cup
- Granulated sugar: 3/4 cup
- Zest of 2 lemons
- Fresh mint leaves, finely chopped: 2 tablespoons
- Fresh mint leaves for garnish (optional)

How to Prepare:

- ✓ The Sweet Beginnings: In the magical pot (saucepan) of beginnings, invite the water and granulated sugar for a dance. Heat this dance floor on a medium tempo, guiding them in their waltz until every sugar crystal vanishes into the embrace of water. This magical potion you've conjured is none other than the 'simple syrup.' Let this potion retreat and cool to the calmness of the room ambiance.
- ✓ A Zesty Twist: When your potion is cool and serene, summon the spirit of sunny lemons—both their zesty peel and their tangy juice. Stir them in, making your potion vibrant and tangy—the elixir of lemon sorbet.

- ✓ The Churning Chronicles: Pour your lemony elixir into the cauldron (ice cream maker) and let it spin and weave its magic, as dictated by its ancient scrolls (manufacturer's instructions). The potion will dance and whirl for approximately two dozen minutes, growing creamier with each spin.
- ✓ A Whiff of Minty Magic: Just as your potion is about to complete its dance, sprinkle in the emerald whispers of freshly chopped mint leaves. Let these leaves waltz in for the finale.
- ✓ The Slumber in Frost: When the dance reaches its crescendo, guide your lemon sorbet into its icy chambers (airtight container) for deep sleep, freezing and dreaming for 4-6 hours. Here, it matures and firms up, readying itself for the grand reveal.
- ✓ The Enchanted Feast: At the hour of dessert, awaken the Lemon Sorbet with Mint from its chambers, enchantingly dolloping it into mystical bowls or magical glasses. Crown with a fresh mint leaf and let the magic unfold on your taste buds!

Nutritional Info: Calories: 162 kcal, Carb: 42g, Sugars: 39g, Protein: 0.5g, Fat: 0g, Sodium: 2mg, Fiber: 0.6g

16. Peanut Butter and Banana Sushi Rolls

(Persons: 2 | Ready in: 10 minutes)

Necessary Items:

- Large whole-wheat tortillas: 2
- Ripe bananas: 2
- Peanut butter (or almond butter): 4 tablespoons
- Honey: 2 tablespoons
- Granola: 1/4 cup
- Ground cinnamon: 1/4 teaspoon
- Fresh berries (strawberries, blueberries, or raspberries) for garnish (optional)

How to Prepare:

- ✓ Lay out the whole-wheat tortillas on a clean, flat surface.
- ✓ In a small microwave-safe bowl, warm the peanut butter (or almond butter) for about 20-30 seconds until it becomes easier to drizzle.
- ✓ Drizzle the warmed peanut butter evenly over each tortilla.
- ✓ Drizzle 1 tablespoon of honey over each tortilla, distributing it evenly.
- ✓ Place a ripe banana on each tortilla, positioning it near the edge closest to you.
- ✓ Sprinkle 2 tablespoons of granola on top of each banana.
- ✓ Add a pinch of ground cinnamon over the granola for extra flavor.
- ✓ Carefully roll up the tortillas, starting from the edge closest to you, and tuck in the sides as you go to create a sushi roll shape.
- ✓ Using a sharp knife, slice each roll into bite-sized pieces, resembling sushi rolls.
- ✓ Optional: Garnish with fresh berries for added color and flavor.

Nutritional Info: Calories: 376 kcal, Carbohydrates: 65g, Sugars: 31g, Protein: 9g, Fat: 11g, Sodium: 272mg, Fiber: 8g

17. Pecan Pie Energy Balls

(Persons: 12-15 energy balls | Ready in: 15 minutes)

Necessary Items:

- Pecans: 1 cup
- Pitted dates: 1 cup
- Rolled oats: 1/4 cup
- Shredded coconut: 1/4 cup
- Vanilla extract: 1 teaspoon
- Ground cinnamon: 1/2 teaspoon
- A pinch of salt
- Water (if needed): 1-2 tablespoons

How to Prepare:

- ✓ Place the pecans in a food processor and pulse until they are finely chopped but not turned into a paste.
- ✓ Add the pitted dates, rolled oats, shredded coconut, vanilla extract, ground cinnamon, and a pinch of salt to the food processor.
- ✓ Pulse the mixture until it starts to come together and forms a sticky dough. If the mixture seems too dry, add 1-2 tablespoons of water and pulse again until well combined.
- ✓ Stop the food processor and scrape down the sides as needed to ensure all ingredients are evenly mixed.
- ✓ Once the mixture resembles a sticky dough, it's ready to be rolled into energy balls.
- ✓ Take small portions of the mixture and roll them between your hands to form compact balls. The size can vary depending on your preference, but aim for 1 to 1.5 inches in diameter.
- ✓ Place the pecan pie energy balls on a parchment paper-lined tray or plate.
- ✓ Optional: You can roll the energy balls in additional shredded coconut or finely chopped pecans for extra flavor and texture.
- ✓ Refrigerate the energy balls for at least 30 minutes to firm them up.
- ✓ Once chilled, transfer them to an airtight container and store them in the refrigerator for up to two weeks.

Nutritional Info: Calories: 119 kcal, Carbohydrates: 15g, Sugars: 10g, Protein: 2g, Fat: 6g, Sodium: 1mg, Fiber: 2g

18. Mixed Berry Yogurt Parfait

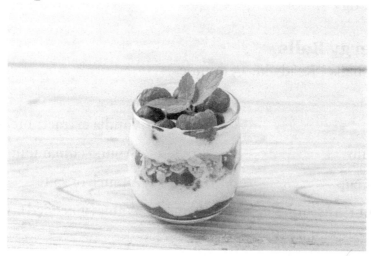

(Persons: 2 | Ready in: 10 minutes)

Necessary Items:

- Greek yogurt (plain or vanilla flavored): 1 cup
- Mixed berries (strawberries, blueberries, raspberries, or your choice): 1 cup
- Granola: 1/2 cup
- Honey or maple syrup (optional for added sweetness): 2 tablespoons
- Fresh mint leaves for garnish (optional)

How to Prepare:

- ✓ Wash and prepare the mixed berries. If using strawberries, remove the stems and slice them.
- ✓ In a bowl, mix the Greek yogurt with honey or maple syrup if you prefer a sweeter yogurt layer. Adjust the sweetness to your taste.
- ✓ Take two serving glasses or bowls.
- ✓ Start by layering the bottom of each glass with a spoonful of Greek yogurt.
- ✓ Add a layer of mixed berries on top of the yogurt.
- ✓ Sprinkle a layer of granola over the berries. You can use store-bought granola or make your own.
- ✓ Repeat the layers - yogurt, berries, and granola - until the glasses are filled.
- ✓ Finish with a dollop of yogurt on the top layer and garnish with a few fresh berries and mint leaves if desired.
- ✓ Serve immediately or refrigerate until ready to eat.

Nutritional Info: Calories: 250 kcal, Carbohydrates: 43g, Sugars: 19g, Protein: 13g, Fat: 4g, Fiber: 6g, Calcium: 150mg, Vitamin C: 35mg

60-Day Meal Plan: 16:8 (16 hours fasting, 8 hours eating)

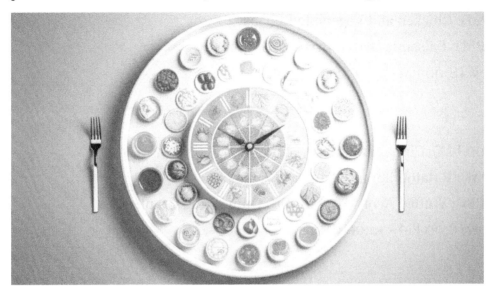

Week 1-2 (Adaptation Phase)

During the first two weeks, women should gradually adjust to intermittent fasting.

Day 1

Breakfast (12:00 PM): Chocolate Banana Smoothie

Lunch (3:00 PM): Teriyaki Salmon with Steamed Broccoli

Dinner (6:00 PM): Creamy Tomato Basil Soup

Fasting Window (8:00 PM - 12:00 PM next day)

Day 2

Breakfast (12:00 PM): Spinach and Mushroom Omelette

Lunch (3:00 PM): Roasted Red Pepper Hummus Wrap

Dinner (6:00 PM): Garlic Butter Shrimp Scampi

Fasting Window (8:00 PM - 12:00 PM next day)

Day 3

Breakfast (12:00 PM): Pumpkin Spice Oatmeal

Lunch (3:00 PM): Seared Tofu with Peanut Sauce

Dinner (6:00 PM): Spinach and Mushroom Stuffed Pork Tenderloin

Fasting Window (8:00 PM - 12:00 PM next day)

Day 4

Breakfast (12:00 PM): Nut Butter and Banana Sandwich

Lunch (3:00 PM): Chicken and Vegetable Kebabs

Dinner (6:00 PM): Balsamic Glazed Brussels Sprouts

Fasting Window (8:00 PM - 12:00 PM next day)

Day 5

Breakfast (12:00 PM): Cinnamon Raisin Toast

Lunch (3:00 PM): Ratatouille with Quinoa

Dinner (6:00 PM): Stuffed Acorn Squash with Quinoa and Cranberries

Fasting Window (8:00 PM - 12:00 PM next day)

Day 6

Breakfast (12:00 PM): Fruit and Nut Muffins

Lunch (3:00 PM): Lemon Garlic Shrimp Skewers

Dinner (6:00 PM): Garlic-Herb Roasted Cod

Fasting Window (8:00 PM - 12:00 PM next day)

Day 7

Breakfast (12:00 PM): Sweet Potato and Black Bean Tacos

Lunch (3:00 PM): Thai-Inspired Vegetable Curry

Dinner (6:00 PM): Creamy Tomato Basil Soup

Fasting Window (8:00 PM - 12:00 PM next day)

Day 8

Breakfast (12:00 PM): Cinnamon Raisin Toast

Lunch (3:00 PM): Zucchini Noodles with Pesto

Dinner (6:00 PM): Garlic Butter Shrimp Scampi

Fasting Window (8:00 PM - 12:00 PM next day)

Day 9

Breakfast (12:00 PM): Egg Muffins

Lunch (3:00 PM): Roasted Beet and Walnut Salad with Citrus Dressing

Dinner (6:00 PM): Spinach and Mushroom Stuffed Pork Tenderloin

Fasting Window (8:00 PM - 12:00 PM next day)

Day 10

Breakfast (12:00 PM): Apricot Almond Bites

Lunch (3:00 PM): Moroccan Spiced Chickpea Stew

Dinner (6:00 PM): Balsamic Glazed Brussels Sprouts

Fasting Window (8:00 PM - 12:00 PM next day)

Day 11

Breakfast (12:00 PM): Nutty Trail Mix

Lunch (3:00 PM): Lemon Rosemary Grilled Swordfish

Dinner (6:00 PM): Stuffed Acorn Squash with Quinoa and Cranberries

Fasting Window (8:00 PM - 12:00 PM next day)

Day 12

Breakfast (12:00 PM): Quinoa Breakfast Bowl

Lunch (3:00 PM): Pesto Spaghetti Squash with Cherry Tomatoes

Dinner (6:00 PM): Garlic-Herb Roasted Cod with Cherry Tomatoes

Fasting Window (8:00 PM - 12:00 PM next day)

Day 13

Breakfast (12:00 PM): Cherry Almond Smoothie

Lunch (3:00 PM): Walnut-Crusted Turkey Cutlets

Dinner (6:00 PM): Grilled Lemon Herb Tofu Steaks

Fasting Window (8:00 PM - 12:00 PM next day)

Day 14

Breakfast (12:00 PM): Caramelized Onion and Goat Cheese Frittata

Lunch (3:00 PM): Cabbage Rolls with Ground Turkey and Rice

Dinner (6:00 PM): Herb-Crusted Pork Loin with Apple Chutney

Fasting Window (8:00 PM - 12:00 PM next day)

Tips for Women Over 70

- **Balanced Nutrition:** Focus on a well-balanced diet rich in whole foods. Include plenty of colorful fruits and vegetables, lean proteins, whole grains, and healthy fats in your meals.

- **Calcium-Rich Foods:** As bone health becomes increasingly important with age, prioritize calcium-rich foods like low-fat dairy, fortified plant-based milk, leafy greens, and canned fish with bones to support bone strength.

- **Protein Intake:** Ensure you're getting enough protein to maintain muscle mass. Include sources like lean meats, poultry, fish, beans, lentils, and Greek yogurt in your meals.

Shopping Advice

- **Shop the Perimeter:** In the grocery store, focus on the perimeter where fresh produce, lean meats, dairy, and whole grains are usually located. This can help you make healthier choices.

- **Read Labels:** Pay attention to food labels, especially for added sugars, sodium, and saturated fats. Opt for products with minimal additives and preservatives.

- **Buy Fresh and Frozen:** Fresh fruits and vegetables are excellent choices, but frozen options can be just as nutritious and have a longer shelf life.

Week 3-4 (Adjustment Phase)

By Weeks 3-4, women should be adjusting well to intermittent fasting.

Day 15

Breakfast (12:00 PM): Herb-Crusted Pork Loin with Apple Chutney

Lunch (3:00 PM): Greek Lemon Chicken Soup (Avgolemono)

Dinner (6:00 PM): Moroccan Spiced Chickpea Stew

Fasting Window (8:00 PM - 12:00 PM next day)

Day 16

Breakfast (12:00 PM): Pesto Spaghetti Squash with Cherry Tomatoes

Lunch (3:00 PM): Sweet Potato and Black Bean Tacos

Dinner (6:00 PM): Creamy Pumpkin and Sage Risotto

Fasting Window (8:00 PM - 12:00 PM next day)

Day 17

Breakfast (12:00 PM): Walnut-Crusted Turkey Cutlets

Lunch (3:00 PM): Sesame-Ginger Salmon with Bok Choy

Dinner (6:00 PM): Coconut Curry Butternut Squash Soup

Fasting Window (8:00 PM - 12:00 PM next day)

Day 18

Breakfast (12:00 PM): Grilled Lemon Herb Tofu Steaks

Lunch (3:00 PM): Cabbage Rolls with Ground Turkey and Rice

Dinner (6:00 PM): Pomegranate Glazed Salmon with Roasted Brussels Sprouts

Fasting Window (8:00 PM - 12:00 PM next day)

Day 19

Breakfast (12:00 PM): Stuffed Bell Peppers with Quinoa and Feta

Lunch (3:00 PM): Mediterranean Tuna and White Bean Salad

Dinner (6:00 PM): Stuffed Acorn Squash with Quinoa and Cranberries

Fasting Window (8:00 PM - 12:00 PM next day)

Day 20

Breakfast (12:00 PM): Cauliflower and Broccoli Casserole with Cheese

Lunch (3:00 PM): Caramelized Onion and Goat Cheese Frittata

Dinner (6:00 PM): Zesty Cucumber and Avocado Gazpacho

Fasting Window (8:00 PM - 12:00 PM next day)

Day 21

Breakfast (12:00 PM): Mango and Shrimp Salad with Chili-Lime Dressing

Lunch (3:00 PM): Thai-Inspired Vegetable Curry

Dinner (6:00 PM): Creamy Tomato Basil Soup

Fasting Window (8:00 PM - 12:00 PM next day)

Day 22

Breakfast (12:00 PM): Mexican Cauliflower Rice Bowl

Lunch (3:00 PM): Spinach and Artichoke Stuffed Chicken Thighs

Dinner (6:00 PM): Roasted Beet and Walnut Salad with Citrus Dressing

Fasting Window (8:00 PM - 12:00 PM next day)

Day 23

Breakfast (12:00 PM): Lemon Rosemary Grilled Swordfish

Lunch (3:00 PM): Creamy Pumpkin and Sage Risotto

Dinner (6:00 PM): Pesto Spaghetti Squash with Cherry Tomatoes

Fasting Window (8:00 PM - 12:00 PM next day)

Day 24

Breakfast (12:00 PM): Walnut-Crusted Turkey Cutlets

Lunch (3:00 PM): Sesame-Ginger Salmon with Bok Choy

Dinner (6:00 PM): Coconut Curry Butternut Squash Soup

Fasting Window (8:00 PM - 12:00 PM next day)

Day 25

Breakfast (12:00 PM): Grilled Lemon Herb Tofu Steaks

Lunch (3:00 PM): Cabbage Rolls with Ground Turkey and Rice

Dinner (6:00 PM): Pomegranate Glazed Salmon with Roasted Brussels Sprouts

Fasting Window (8:00 PM - 12:00 PM next day)

Day 26

Breakfast (12:00 PM): Stuffed Bell Peppers with Quinoa and Feta

Lunch (3:00 PM): Mediterranean Tuna and White Bean Salad

Dinner (6:00 PM): Stuffed Acorn Squash with Quinoa and Cranberries

Fasting Window (8:00 PM - 12:00 PM next day)

Day 27

Breakfast (12:00 PM): Cauliflower and Broccoli Casserole with Cheese

Lunch (3:00 PM): Caramelized Onion and Goat Cheese Frittata

Dinner (6:00 PM): Zesty Cucumber and Avocado Gazpacho

Fasting Window (8:00 PM - 12:00 PM next day)

Day 28

Breakfast (12:00 PM): Mango and Shrimp Salad with Chili-Lime Dressing

Lunch (3:00 PM): Thai-Inspired Vegetable Curry

Dinner (6:00 PM): Creamy Tomato Basil Soup

Fasting Window (8:00 PM - 12:00 PM next day)

Tips for Women Over 70

- **Fiber-Rich Foods:** Fiber aids digestion and helps manage weight. Incorporate high-fiber foods like whole grains, oats, beans, and vegetables into your diet.

- **Hydration:** Staying hydrated is crucial. Sip water throughout the day, and consider herbal teas or infused water for variety. Dehydration can sometimes be mistaken for hunger.

- **Healthy Fats:** Include sources of healthy fats, such as avocados, nuts, seeds, and olive oil, to support heart health and cognitive function.

- **Limit Added Sugars:** Minimize your intake of sugary foods and beverages, which can lead to energy spikes and crashes. Opt for natural sweeteners like honey or maple syrup in moderation.

Shopping Advice

- **Choose Whole Grains:** Look for whole grains like brown rice, quinoa, and whole wheat bread instead of refined grains. They provide more nutrients and fiber.

- **Stock up on Healthy Snacks:** Have healthy snacks like nuts, seeds, Greek yogurt, and fresh fruit on hand to prevent reaching for less nutritious options.

- **Limit Processed Foods:** Minimize the purchase of processed and pre-packaged foods, as they often contain unhealthy additives and preservatives.

Week 7-8 (Maintenance Phase)

By Weeks 7-8, women should be fully adapted to intermittent fasting.

Day 29

Breakfast (12:00 PM): Walnut-Crusted Turkey Cutlets

Lunch (3:00 PM): Pomegranate Glazed Salmon with Roasted Brussels Sprouts

Dinner (6:00 PM): Stuffed Bell Peppers with Quinoa and Feta

Fasting Window (8:00 PM - 12:00 PM next day)

Day 30

Breakfast (12:00 PM): Cauliflower and Broccoli Casserole with Cheese

Lunch (3:00 PM): Zesty Cucumber and Avocado Gazpacho

Dinner (6:00 PM): Thai-Inspired Vegetable Curry

Fasting Window (8:00 PM - 12:00 PM next day)

Day 31

Breakfast (12:00 PM): Mango and Shrimp Salad with Chili-Lime Dressing

Lunch (3:00 PM): Creamy Tomato Basil Soup

Dinner (6:00 PM): Spinach and Mushroom Stuffed Pork Tenderloin

Fasting Window (8:00 PM - 12:00 PM next day)

Day 32

Breakfast (12:00 PM): Roasted Beet and Walnut Salad with Citrus Dressing

Lunch (3:00 PM): Coconut Curry Butternut Squash Soup

Dinner (6:00 PM): Lemon Rosemary Grilled Swordfish

Fasting Window (8:00 PM - 12:00 PM next day)

Day 33

Breakfast (12:00 PM): Pesto Spaghetti Squash with Cherry Tomatoes

Lunch (3:00 PM): Caramelized Onion and Goat Cheese Frittata

Dinner (6:00 PM): Garlic-Herb Roasted Cod with Cherry Tomatoes

Fasting Window (8:00 PM - 12:00 PM next day)

Day 34

Breakfast (12:00 PM): Stuffed Acorn Squash with Quinoa and Cranberries

Lunch (3:00 PM): Mediterranean Tuna and White Bean Salad

Dinner (6:00 PM): Zucchini Noodles with Pesto

Fasting Window (8:00 PM - 12:00 PM next day)

Day 35

Breakfast (12:00 PM): Cabbage Rolls with Ground Turkey and Rice

Lunch (3:00 PM): Mexican Cauliflower Rice Bowl

Dinner (6:00 PM): Spinach and Artichoke Stuffed Chicken Thighs

Fasting Window (8:00 PM - 12:00 PM next day)

Day 36

Breakfast (12:00 PM): Pumpkin Spice Oatmeal

Lunch (3:00 PM): Seared Tofu with Peanut Sauce

Dinner (6:00 PM): Spinach and Mushroom Stuffed Pork Tenderloin

Fasting Window (8:00 PM - 12:00 PM next day)

Day 37

Breakfast (12:00 PM): Nut Butter and Banana Sandwich

Lunch (3:00 PM): Chicken and Vegetable Kebabs

Dinner (6:00 PM): Balsamic Glazed Brussels Sprouts

Fasting Window (8:00 PM - 12:00 PM next day)

Day 38

Breakfast (12:00 PM): Cinnamon Raisin Toast

Lunch (3:00 PM): Ratatouille with Quinoa

Dinner (6:00 PM): Stuffed Acorn Squash with Quinoa and Cranberries

Fasting Window (8:00 PM - 12:00 PM next day)

Day 39

Breakfast (12:00 PM): Fruit and Nut Muffins

Lunch (3:00 PM): Lemon Garlic Shrimp Skewers

Dinner (6:00 PM): Garlic-Herb Roasted Cod

Fasting Window (8:00 PM - 12:00 PM next day)

Day 40

Breakfast (12:00 PM): Chocolate Banana Smoothie

Lunch (3:00 PM): Roasted Red Pepper Hummus Wrap

Dinner (6:00 PM): Sweet Potato and Black Bean Tacos

Fasting Window (8:00 PM - 12:00 PM next day)

Day 41

Breakfast (12:00 PM): Spinach and Mushroom Omelette

Lunch (3:00 PM): Teriyaki Salmon with Steamed Broccoli

Dinner (6:00 PM): Caprese Chicken Salad

Fasting Window (8:00 PM - 12:00 PM next day)

Day 42

Breakfast (12:00 PM): Your choice from the provided breakfast recipes.

Lunch (3:00 PM): Your choice from the provided lunch recipes.

Dinner (6:00 PM): Your choice from the provided dinner recipes.

Fasting Window (8:00 PM - 12:00 PM next day)

Tips for Women Over 70

- **Regular Exercise:** Incorporate regular physical activity into your routine. Choose exercises that suit your fitness level, such as walking, yoga, or water aerobics, to maintain strength and flexibility.

- **Bone Health:** Besides calcium, ensure you're getting enough vitamin D, which aids in calcium absorption. Spend time in the sun, eat vitamin D-rich foods like fatty fish and fortified cereals, or consider supplements if advised by your doctor.

- **Medication Management:** If you take medications, be mindful of any fasting requirements. Some medications may need to be taken with food, so discuss this with your healthcare provide

- **Regular Check-ups:** Schedule regular check-ups with your healthcare provider to monitor your health, including blood pressure, cholesterol, and bone density.

Shopping Advice

- **Try Online Shopping:** Online grocery shopping can be convenient, especially if mobility is a concern. Many stores offer delivery or curbside pickup services.

- **Buy in Bulk:** For non-perishable items like beans, whole grains, and canned goods, consider buying in bulk to save money and reduce the need for frequent shopping trips.

<u>Week 9-10 (Optimization Phase)</u>

During Weeks 9-10, women should focus on optimizing their intermittent fasting routine.

Day 43

Breakfast (12:00 PM): Walnut-Crusted Turkey Cutlets

Lunch (3:00 PM): Pomegranate Glazed Salmon with Roasted Brussels Sprouts

Dinner (6:00 PM): Stuffed Bell Peppers with Quinoa and Feta

Fasting Window (8:00 PM - 12:00 PM next day)

Day 44

Breakfast (12:00 PM): Cauliflower and Broccoli Casserole with Cheese

Lunch (3:00 PM): Zesty Cucumber and Avocado Gazpacho

Dinner (6:00 PM): Thai-Inspired Vegetable Curry

Fasting Window (8:00 PM - 12:00 PM next day)

Day 45

Breakfast (12:00 PM): Mango and Shrimp Salad with Chili-Lime Dressing

Lunch (3:00 PM): Creamy Tomato Basil Soup

Dinner (6:00 PM): Spinach and Mushroom Stuffed Pork Tenderloin

Fasting Window (8:00 PM - 12:00 PM next day)

Day 46

Breakfast (12:00 PM): Roasted Beet and Walnut Salad with Citrus Dressing

Lunch (3:00 PM): Coconut Curry Butternut Squash Soup

Dinner (6:00 PM): Lemon Rosemary Grilled Swordfish

Fasting Window (8:00 PM - 12:00 PM next day)

Day 47

Breakfast (12:00 PM): Pesto Spaghetti Squash with Cherry Tomatoes

Lunch (3:00 PM): Caramelized Onion and Goat Cheese Frittata

Dinner (6:00 PM): Garlic-Herb Roasted Cod with Cherry Tomatoes

Fasting Window (8:00 PM - 12:00 PM next day)

Day 48

Breakfast (12:00 PM): Chocolate Banana Smoothie

Lunch (3:00 PM): Roasted Red Pepper Hummus Wrap

Dinner (6:00 PM): Sweet Potato and Black Bean Tacos

Fasting Window (8:00 PM - 12:00 PM next day)

Day 49

Breakfast (12:00 PM): Spinach and Mushroom Omelette

Lunch (3:00 PM): Teriyaki Salmon with Steamed Broccoli

Dinner (6:00 PM): Caprese Chicken Salad

Fasting Window (8:00 PM - 12:00 PM next day)

Day 50

Breakfast (12:00 PM): Your choice from the provided breakfast recipes.

Lunch (3:00 PM): Your choice from the provided lunch recipes.

Dinner (6:00 PM): Your choice from the provided dinner recipes.

Fasting Window (8:00 PM - 12:00 PM next day)

Day 51

Breakfast (12:00 PM): Walnut-Crusted Turkey Cutlets

Lunch (3:00 PM): Pomegranate Glazed Salmon with Roasted Brussels Sprouts

Dinner (6:00 PM): Stuffed Bell Peppers with Quinoa and Feta

Fasting Window (8:00 PM - 12:00 PM next day)

Day 52

Breakfast (12:00 PM): Cauliflower and Broccoli Casserole with Cheese

Lunch (3:00 PM): Zesty Cucumber and Avocado Gazpacho

Dinner (6:00 PM): Thai-Inspired Vegetable Curry

Fasting Window (8:00 PM - 12:00 PM next day)

Day 53

Breakfast (12:00 PM): Mango and Shrimp Salad with Chili-Lime Dressing

Lunch (3:00 PM): Creamy Tomato Basil Soup

Dinner (6:00 PM): Spinach and Mushroom Stuffed Pork Tenderloin

Fasting Window (8:00 PM - 12:00 PM next day)

Day 54

Breakfast (12:00 PM): Roasted Beet and Walnut Salad with Citrus Dressing

Lunch (3:00 PM): Coconut Curry Butternut Squash Soup

Dinner (6:00 PM): Lemon Rosemary Grilled Swordfish

Fasting Window (8:00 PM - 12:00 PM next day)

Day 55

Breakfast (12:00 PM): Pesto Spaghetti Squash with Cherry Tomatoes

Lunch (3:00 PM): Caramelized Onion and Goat Cheese Frittata

Dinner (6:00 PM): Garlic-Herb Roasted Cod with Cherry Tomatoes

Fasting Window (8:00 PM - 12:00 PM next day)

Day 56

Breakfast (12:00 PM): Chocolate Banana Smoothie

Lunch (3:00 PM): Roasted Red Pepper Hummus Wrap

Dinner (6:00 PM): Sweet Potato and Black Bean Tacos

Fasting Window (8:00 PM - 12:00 PM next day)

Day 57

Breakfast (12:00 PM): Spinach and Mushroom Omelette

Lunch (3:00 PM): Teriyaki Salmon with Steamed Broccoli

Dinner (6:00 PM): Caprese Chicken Salad

Fasting Window (8:00 PM - 12:00 PM next day)

Day 58

Breakfast (12:00 PM): Your choice from the provided breakfast recipes.

Lunch (3:00 PM): Your choice from the provided lunch recipes.

Dinner (6:00 PM): Your choice from the provided dinner recipes.

Fasting Window (8:00 PM - 12:00 PM next day)

Day 59

Breakfast (12:00 PM): Walnut-Crusted Turkey Cutlets

Lunch (3:00 PM): Pomegranate Glazed Salmon with Roasted Brussels Sprouts

Dinner (6:00 PM): Stuffed Bell Peppers with Quinoa and Feta

Fasting Window (8:00 PM - 12:00 PM next day)

Day 60 (Final Day)

Breakfast (12:00 PM): Cauliflower and Broccoli Casserole with Cheese

Lunch (3:00 PM): Zesty Cucumber and Avocado Gazpacho

Dinner (6:00 PM): Thai-Inspired Vegetable Curry

Congratulations On Completing The 60-Day Intermittent Fasting Meal Plan!

By now, you should have adapted to this eating pattern and experienced its potential benefits. Remember to continue making mindful food choices and listening to your body's needs.

Guided Intermittent Fasting Tracker

Name:

Start Date of Tracking:

Intermittent Fasting Goal:

Fasting Window

Record the start and end times of your daily fasting window. You can also note any variations in fasting duration or days when you followed a different fasting window.

Day 1
Fasting Start Time:
Fasting End Time:
Notes:
...

Day 2
Fasting Start Time:
Fasting End Time:
Notes:

Nutrition Intake

Log the meals and snacks you consume during the eating window. Pay attention to portion sizes and the quality of foods you choose.

Day 1

Meal 1:

Meal 2:

Snack:

Notes:

...

Day 2

Meal 1:

Meal 2:

Snack:

Notes:

Non-Scale Victories

Every day, write down the non-scale victories you experienced thanks to intermittent fasting. These could include improved digestion, reduced cravings, enhanced focus, or healthier skin.

Day 1

Non-Scale Victory:

Notes:

...

Day 2

Non-Scale Victory:

Notes:

Energy and Well-being

Monitor your energy levels and overall well-being throughout the day. Take note of any variations or changes you noticed.

Day 1

Energy Levels:

General Well-being:

Notes:

...

Day 2

Energy Levels:

General Well-being:

Notes:

Physical Changes

Occasionally, take time to evaluate any physical changes. These may include weight loss, measurements, or body composition.

Day 1

Weight:

Measurements:

Body Composition:

Notes:

...

Day 2

Weight:

Measurements:

Body Composition:

Notes

Guided Roadmap for Intermittent Fasting

These guides will help the reader track their intermittent fasting progress in a structured and mindful way. Remind them to be patient with themselves, as every body responds differently. The key is to tailor intermittent fasting to their individual needs and experiment until they find the best routine for their journey.

Step 1: Choose Your Tracker

Select the tracking method that suits you best: pen and paper, mobile app, or smartwatch/fitness tracker.

Step 2: Clear Goals

Clearly define your intermittent fasting goals, such as weight loss, improved energy, or better mental clarity.

Step 3: Fasting Windows

Record the start and end times of your daily fasting window and experiment with different fasting windows to find the one that works best for you.

Step 4: Mindful Eating

Monitor what you eat during the eating windows, ensuring you make nutritious and balanced choices.

Step 5: Non-Scale Victories

Recognize victories unrelated to the scale, such as better sleep, reduced heartburn, or an improved mood.

Step 6: Energy and Well-being

Be mindful of your energy levels throughout the day and how intermittent fasting impacts your overall well-being.

Step 7: Physical Changes

Occasionally evaluate any physical changes, but remember that progress may be gradual and vary from person to person.

Step 8: Reflection and Adaptation

Weekly, reflect on your progress and adapt your intermittent fasting routine based on results and personal needs.

Step 9: Celebrate Success

Celebrate your successes and small victories along the intermittent fasting journey to keep motivation high.

Conclusion

This comprehensive guide, "Intermittent Fasting For Women Over 70," has taken you on a transformative journey tailored to the unique needs and aspirations of women in this age group. Throughout these pages, we've explored the incredible potential of intermittent fasting, providing you with the knowledge, tools, and inspiration to embrace this lifestyle fully.

We unlocked the power of intermittent fasting, delving into its fundamental principles and the science behind its remarkable benefits. We tailored intermittent fasting methods to suit the needs of women over 70, offering expert guidance on initiating and sustaining this dietary approach safely. We recognized that navigating the aging process comes with its own set of challenges and opportunities. We explored the physiological changes women experience after 70 and how fasting can address these challenges. We encouraged you to integrate intermittent fasting into your lifestyle, building confidence along the way. Moreover, we discussed dietary options, supplements, and resources for success, even considering the integration of traditional medicine and natural remedies. Physical activity was not overlooked, as we highlighted the synergy between intermittent fasting and exercise. A 30-day exercise plan designed for women over 70 was included to promote holistic wellness and optimal aging. Moreover, we guided you in discovering reliable resources, connecting with like-minded individuals, involving loved ones, and enlisting supportive friends on your fasting journey. Building a support system is invaluable as you embrace this transformative lifestyle. Our journey through this book wouldn't be complete without a delectable array of recipes tailored to intermittent fasting. From satisfying breakfast options to delicious lunches and dinners, and even snacks and desserts, we've ensured that your meals can be both nutritious and enjoyable. As you've ventured through the 60-day meal plan, you've learned the art of intermittent fasting, following a 16:8 schedule, and tracking your progress with the provided guided intermittent fasting tracker and roadmap.

Intermittent fasting is not just about changing your diet; it's about changing your life. It's a journey of self-discovery, empowerment, and rejuvenation. We hope that the knowledge and resources shared in this book have equipped you to embark on this journey with confidence and enthusiasm. Remember, age is but a number, and it's never too late to embrace a healthier, more vibrant you. Celebrate your non-scale victories, listen to your body, and continue exploring the endless possibilities of intermittent fasting. Your path may be unique, but the benefits of improved health, increased vitality, and a more fulfilling life are within your reach.

Made in the USA
Las Vegas, NV
11 April 2024